# Atopic Dermatitis - Bridging the Gap between Clinical Science and Practical Care

*Edited by Mohammed Sami Al Abadie*

Published in London, United Kingdom

Atopic Dermatitis - Bridging the Gap between Clinical Science and Practical Care
http://dx.doi.org/10.5772/intechopen.1007245
Edited by Mohammed Sami Al Abadie

Contributors
Abdullah Ahmed Alhejaily, Amr Molla, Aylin Turel Ermertcan, Mohammed Alraddadi, Muhammed Ali Mergen, Nadir Omar, Noura Elgharably, Tubanur Cetinarslan, Zinah Sharara



First published in London, United Kingdom, 2026 by IntechOpen
IntechOpen is the global imprint of INTECHOPEN LIMITED, registered in England and Wales, registration number: 11086078, 167-169 Great Portland Street, London, W1W 5PF, United Kingdom

For EU product safety concerns: IN TECH d.o.o., Prolaz Marije Krucifikse Kozulić 3, 51000 Rijeka, Croatia, info@intechopen.com or visit our website at intechopen.com.

British Library Cataloguing-in-Publication Data
A catalogue record for this book is available from the British Library

Atopic Dermatitis - Bridging the Gap between Clinical Science and Practical Care
Edited by Mohammed Sami Al Abadie
p. cm.
Print ISBN 978-1-83635-010-1
Online ISBN 978-1-83635-009-5
eBook (PDF) ISBN 978-1-83635-011-8

If disposing of this product, please recycle the paper responsibly.

# Meet the editor

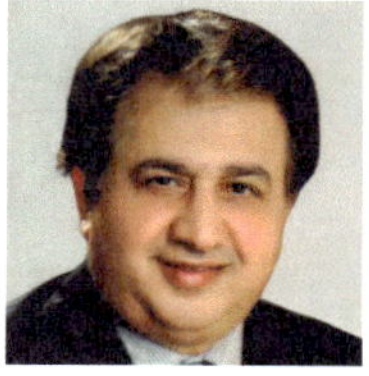

Professor Mohammed Sami Al Abadie is Clinical Professor of Dermatology at the University of Wolverhampton and serves as Clinical Director and Consultant Dermatologist at North Cumbria Integrated NHS Foundation Trust, United Kingdom. With over three decades of experience in dermatology, he has contributed extensively to clinical practice, academic teaching, and research innovation. Professor Al Abadie is a Fellow of the Royal Colleges of Physicians of London, Edinburgh, and Glasgow, and holds a Ph.D. in Dermatology from the University of Sheffield. Internationally recognised for his leadership and expertise, he has published widely and is Editor-in-Chief of the *International Journal of Clinical and Experimental Dermatology*.

# Contents

# Preface

*Atopic Dermatitis – Bridging the Gap between Clinical Science and Practical Care* brings together clinical experience and current understanding of atopic dermatitis (AD) to provide an accessible overview for specialists and general practitioners alike. The book aims to close the divide between research knowledge and everyday patient care, helping clinicians translate advances in science into improved clinical outcomes.

Atopic dermatitis is a complex, multifactorial condition that affects patients across all age groups, but most commonly begins in childhood. It has significant links with allergies, asthma, and other atopic disorders, and continues to pose challenges for effective management. This volume presents a balanced view of the condition, from pathophysiology and diagnosis to treatment and long-term care, with emphasis on practical, evidence-based approaches.

The chapters collectively explore key areas including disease mechanisms, allergic associations, and therapeutic strategies. Special attention is given to the management of atopic dermatitis in children, where early recognition and appropriate intervention can have lifelong benefits. The book also discusses conventional and modern treatments, highlighting the growing role of biologic agents, personalized care, and multidisciplinary collaboration.

By integrating clinical insight with recent developments, this volume aims to support healthcare professionals in delivering holistic and patient-centred care. We hope it encourages further understanding and collaboration in the management of atopic dermatitis and related allergic conditions.

We express our sincere gratitude to all contributing authors and reviewers for their valuable input, and to the IntechOpen editorial team for their professional support throughout the publication process.

**Mohammed Sami Al Abadie**
Professor,
Clinical Professor of Dermatology,
Clinical Director and Consultant Dermatologist,
University of Wolverhampton,
Wolverhampton, England

North Cumbria NHS integrated Trust,
United Kingdom

Chapter 1

# Atopic Dermatitis and Allergy

*Noura Elgharably and Nadir Omar*


## Abstract

Atopic dermatitis (AD) is a common, chronic inflammatory skin condition characterised by relapsing, erythematous, itchy, and dry skin. Its pathogenesis involves a dysfunctional epidermal barrier, immune dysregulation, and environmental factors. Key factors contributing to barrier impairment include filaggrin mutations, imbalanced proteases, and abnormal lipid levels. This chapter will delve into the multifaceted relationship between AD and allergy, encompassing food allergy, aeroallergens, and other triggers, with strong genetic predisposition and family history being significant risk factors. AD is closely linked to other atopic diseases including allergic rhinitis and food allergy. Combined, these form the atopic triad. We will explore the dual allergen exposure hypothesis, emphasising how compromised skin barrier function in AD patients facilitates antigen penetration and promotes transcutaneous sensitisation to environmental allergens. While diagnostic approaches for allergies have evolved, the oral food challenge (OFC) remains the gold standard for confirming food allergies. Early and regular introduction of common food allergens in infants shows promise in prevention, contrasting with limited benefits from general emollient use for AD prevention. Advancements in genetic research, biomarker identification, microbiome studies, identifying genetic loci, and addressing skin dysbiosis, particularly *Staphylococcus aureus* overgrowth, offer opportunities for effective and personalised management approaches to improve patient outcomes and quality of life.


**Keywords:** skin barrier dysfunction, allergens, atopic march, immune dysregulation, food allergy

## 1. Introduction

Atopic dermatitis (AD), often known as atopic eczema, is a common, chronic, inflammatory skin condition. Although predominantly in children, AD can occur in any age group. The relapsing and remitting nature of atopic dermatitis is characterised by erythematous, itchy, and dry skin, often localised but not limited to the flexural regions [1, 2].

The pathogenesis involves a disrupted epidermal barrier, immune dysregulation, and environmental interactions [3]. The epidermis is the outermost layer of this and contains epithelial cells, immune cells, and microbes. These provide both a physical and functional barrier to the skin and prevent the penetration of environmental, irritant, and food allergens. Multiple factors can disrupt the skin's barrier including immune dysregulation, filaggrin mutations, and imbalance in skin's microbial composition.

AD has been closely linked to atopic disease. Early onset or severe subtypes often precedes the development of other allergic conditions including food allergy, asthma, and rhinitis [4]. The combination of atopic dermatitis, asthma, and allergic rhinitis constitute the atopic triad. Atopy refers to the genetic tendency to overproduce immunoglobulin E antibodies (IgE) when exposed to different irritants including pollen, house dust mites, and food allergens. Personal and family history of atopic disease are significant risk factors [5]. Having a family history of atopic disease is a strong risk factor for the development of AD, with approximately 70% of patients affected. The likelihood of AD is three times higher if one patient has atopic disease or five times higher with both parents [6].

## 2. Immune dysregulation and atopic dermatitis

The pathogenesis of AD involves the complex interaction between a dysfunctional epidermal barrier and immune dysregulation.

Genetics play a significant role in AD with genetic predisposition evident and found to be of higher concordance rate in monozygotic twins, 80%, compared to 30% in dizygotic twins [7]. A parental history of AD is also a stronger risk factor for developing the condition than a family history of asthma or allergic rhinitis [6, 8].

A key component in AD pathogenesis is the compromised function of the stratum corneum. The most significant genetic factor for this is mutation in the filaggrin gene, resulting in filaggrin deficiency [9]. Filaggrin is an essential intracellular protein which helps aggregate keratin filaments in the stratum corneum and strengthens the skin barrier. Additionally, the breakdown products of filaggrin provide hydrating factors for the skin. Therefore, a deficiency in filaggrin alters the aggregation of keratin filaments at the skin barrier and skin hydration, resulting in epidermal barrier dysfunction [10, 11].

Another factor which contributes to a defected barrier is imbalanced proteases. An increase in proteases kallikrein 5 and 7, coupled with a decrease in inhibitors leads to excessive breakdown of the proteins responsible for epidermal barrier integrity [12]. Additionally, abnormal ceramide levels in the epidermis contribute to lipid imbalance. Lamellar bodies are required to transport essential lipids to the stratum corneum. Filaggrin deficiency results in defective secretion of this lipid component from lamellar bodies, further compromising the barrier's integrity. Ultimately, a defective epidermal barrier allows various antigens to penetrate the skin, leading to an immune response in AD [10–12].

### 2.1 Immune dysregulation

AD involves a complex interplay of immune responses. When antigens penetrate the compromised skin barrier, dendritic cells present them to naive T cells, initiating a Type 4 hypersensitivity response that drives the Th2 immune pathway [13, 14].

IgE antibodies are a hallmark of allergic reactions and play a role in AD. After exposure to an antigen, IgE antibodies form and bind to mast cells and basophils.

Th2 cytokines, particularly Interleukin 4 (IL-4) and Interleukin 13 (IL-13), are dominant in this pathway. These downregulate crucial proteins like filaggrin, loricrin, and involucrin, all vital for skin moisture retention. Filaggrin mutations are linked to earlier onset and more severe disease. IL-4 also weakens the skin's defences by decreasing cutaneous defence cells and increasing bacterial adhesion molecules, facilitating Staphylococcus aureus (*S. aureus*) colonisation. Keratinocytes further amplify the Th2 response by producing cytokines like IL-1, IL-25, and IL-33. Thymic stromal lymphopoietin (TSLP) also plays a critical role in promoting the Th2 response and contributing to the intense itching associated with AD [14].

As AD progresses to its chronic phase, IL-5 becomes more predominant, and other adaptive immune responses, including Th1, Th17, and Th22 pathways, also are present. Beyond adaptive immunity, innate immune dysregulation is also central to AD. The innate lymphoid cell increases significantly in AD patients and further fuels the Th2 response [15].

The skin microbiome represents a diverse community of bacteria, fungi, and viruses that play a role in epidermal homeostasis. Over 90% of AD patients have skin colonised by *S. aureus*, compared to only 5% of unaffected individuals. During AD flares, bacterial diversity decreases, and the microbiome proportion of *S. aureus* can increase from 35–90%. This *S. aureus* can produce superantigens that further promote the Th2 response. The combined effects of a dysfunctional epidermal barrier, a skewed Th2 immune response, and an altered skin microbiome led to a vicious cycle with increased skin inflammation and heightened transepidermal water loss, resulting in the characteristic dry, inflamed skin of AD [13–15].

To summarise, a compromised epidermal barrier, due to factors like decreased filaggrin, increased proteases, and abnormal lipids, allows antigens to penetrate the skin. These antigens are then presented by dendritic cells to naive T cells, sparking a dominant Th2 response. Cytokines like IL-4, IL-5, and IL-13 further exacerbate this by downregulating filaggrin in the stratum corneum. The release of IgE, binding to Langerhans cells, further amplifies antigen presentation and perpetuates this Th2-skewed environment. This complex process, compounded by an increase in innate lymphoid cells and enhanced *S. aureus* colonisation (with its superantigen production), leads to the chronic inflammation, increased transepidermal water loss, and dryness characteristic of AD.

## 3. Common allergens and triggers in atopic dermatitis

Allergens are defined as environmental or airborne substances which can trigger an allergic reaction. Most commonly linked with atopic dermatitis are aeroallergens, such as house dust mites, mould spores, pet dander, cigarette smoke and pollen, or food allergens such as dairy, nuts, egg, fish/seafood and wheat, or contact allergens such as latex, formaldehyde, and nickel. Contact allergens can also be referred to as haptans which are molecules which become allergenic when bound to proteins in the skin and form a foreign immune complex.

Early and regular introduction of common food allergens in children, such as peanut and egg, have been recommended in complementary feeding regimes from 6 months of age to support the prevention of such allergies in later life. The dual allergen hypothesis was first proposed by Lack et al. in the early 2000s and explored the early introduction of food allergens and its effect on allergy prevention or determination [4]. This contrasted the theories at the time; however, Lack et al. suggested early and regular consumption of these food types would aid the immune response and result in tolerance to these potential allergens. This hypothesis was strengthened by the learning early about peanuts (LEAP) project which demonstrated that early introduction of peanut containing foods reduced later risk of peanut allergy compared to those who avoided peanuts or peanut containing foods completely

[16]. Many other studies have also supported this hypothesis, and there has been no association with maternal peanut consumption during pregnancy or lactation, and sensitisation [17].

Various environmental triggers and harsh irritants such as humidity, sweat, certain fragrances, soaps, stress, and temperature changes can all compromise the skin's barrier and further exacerbate AD symptoms.

An impaired skin barrier in AD allows for penetration of allergens and has been linked to the development of food allergy. When allergens enter the skin, they are taken by dendritic cells and presented to naïve CD4+ T cells. These T cells are activated and produce Th2 cytokines which signal to B cells to produce allergen-specific IgE. This sequence leads to common IgE-mediated food allergy symptoms such as erythema, itchiness, urticaria, and occasionally respiratory issues [15]. This cycle weakens the skin's barrier further and results in a dry, itchy surface which is susceptible to additional reactions.

The implications of a dysfunctional skin barrier are highlighted by a study which looked at the quantities of household peanut protein and found a significantly higher risk of peanut sensitisation in children with filaggrin mutations [18]. This research revealed that early life exposure to allergens through an impaired skin barrier causes Th2 immune response skewing towards innate cytokines, in particular the allergic type Th2 cells (IL-4, IL-5, IL-13). This consequently leads to an IgE-mediated response and food allergy [18]. Thus, we can infer that prevention of allergens from crossing the skin barrier can reduce the likelihood of food allergies and other allergic conditions related to the atopic triad. Additionally, early and regular oral introduction of the allergen can promote immune tolerance and limit the effects of environmental exposure.

## 4. Diagnosing allergies in atopic dermatitis and management strategies

Radioallergosorbent testing (RAST) analyzes the blood for certain IgE antibodies to known or suspected antigens and can be used to confirm specific allergens that cause a hypersensitivity response [19, 20].

RAST is a simple, reliable test for IgE antibodies that is very useful for in vitro diagnosis of atopic allergy on a routine basis [20]. Although advances in immunoassay technologies have led to the widespread adoption of more sensitive, automated platforms, RAST remains historically and methodologically significant [20, 21].

RAST was introduced in the late 1960s as a novel method to detect allergen-specific immunoglobulin E (IgE) antibodies in patient serum. The test quickly gained recognition for its ability to objectively quantify sensitisation to specific allergens without requiring direct skin exposure, thus avoiding the risks of severe cutaneous or systemic reactions often associated with in vivo testing procedures [20, 21]. RAST represented a major technological advancement at the time, offering a reproducible, laboratory-based alternative to skin prick and intradermal testing.

The solid-phase immunoassays based on the enzyme linked immunosorbent assay (ELISA) model for routine immunochemical diagnostics, including the measurement of specific IgE levels, were available as early as the 1970s [20, 21]. Initially, radioimmunoassays (radioallergosorbent test, RAST) were used. RAST tests consisted of immobilising allergen extracts on activated paper discs to bind specific IgE from the patient's serum. Paper discs were the solid phase of the RAST test.

Radiolabels were used to detect allergen/specific IgE immune complexes in RAST tests [22].

RAST has long been employed in the diagnostic workup of multiple allergic diseases. Allergic sensitisation not only covers clinically apparent allergies, but indicates a prognostic factor for later allergies, even in adulthood [23]. RAST testing is a valuable clinical test that should be considered early to investigate patients with AD for relevant allergens that may be exacerbating their symptoms and causing resistance to first line treatment [23, 24].

Despite its diagnostic relevance, RAST has largely been replaced in modern laboratories by enzyme-based immunoassays such as ELISAs, fluorescent enzyme immunoassays (FEIAs), and chemiluminescent assays [25]. These platforms offer enhanced analytical sensitivity, improved reproducibility, and shorter turnaround times, thereby aligning more effectively with the operational needs of contemporary diagnostic laboratories [25, 26].

The oral food challenge (OFC) remains the gold standard available in both research and clinical practice [27]. This organised diagnostic technique is necessary to determine whether a patient has a true food allergy, as opposed to a sensitisation without clinical symptoms [27, 28].

OFCs are essential for both the initial diagnosis and determining whether a food allergy has been resolved because they enable direct observation of the body's reaction to a food. This is especially important for children, who frequently outgrow allergies to common antigens like cow's milk, eggs, wheat, and soy [29].

OFCs need to be conducted with appropriate safety measures in place considering the possibility for adverse responses. It is believed that safe delivery requires clinical settings that are prepared to manage anaphylaxis and personnel who have received emergency response and allergen dosage protocol training [29, 30]. The 2024 American Academy of Allergy, Asthma and Immunology and The European Academy of Allergy and Clinical Immunology (AAAAI–EAACI) update provides comprehensive instructions for carrying out these challenges, such as gradual dose escalation, typically semi-logarithmic increases spaced 20 to 30 minutes apart, and well-defined criteria for test continuation, observation, or termination based on clinical signs [30, 31].

Modern diagnostic techniques including the basophil activation test (BAT) and component-resolved diagnostics (CRD) have become useful supplements. These techniques provide better specificity for individual allergens, but they are not yet a replacement for OFCs, which are still required when clinical uncertainty continues [32]. Sensitisation test findings, a thorough clinical history, and the patient's risk profile are usually taken into consideration when deciding whether to move on with a food challenge in practice [30, 32].

In summary, OFCs play a critical role in the diagnosis and continuing treatment of food allergies. By providing tangible evidence of clinical reactivity, they serve to avoid sensitised persons from being mislabelled as allergic and ensure that elimination diets are only used when absolutely necessary.

While the oral food challenge remains the gold standard for diagnosing food allergies, a well-documented clinical history plays an essential role in guiding test interpretation and clinical decision-making [33].

Clinical history is also indispensable in identifying non-IgE-mediated food allergies, which often elude standard allergy testing and require structured elimination diets followed by supervised reintroduction for confirmation [33, 34]. Furthermore, clinical evaluation helps determine when an OFC is warranted, assess the risk of reaction, and inform individualised care based on factors such as age, symptom pattern, and prior exposures [33, 34].

## 5. Emerging concepts

### 5.1 Prevention

Early preventative strategies, particularly the early introduction of allergenic foods in infants with known AD, have shown promise in the prevention of food allergy.

Prevention strategies have focused on early infancy periods, research studies have explored the application of regular emollients and this effect on AD and FA.

The BEEP study, which looked at regular emollient application from birth and its role in prevention of eczema, found no clinical significance of regular emollient application in the prevention of eczema [35]. There was evidence for increased skin infections with emollient application and no correlation with regular emollient use in the delay, suppression or prevention of eczema at 2 years [35]. It is thought that the higher risk of infection stemmed from a disrupted skin microbiome, an increased number of pathogens introduced to the infant's skin during application, and emollients altering the skin's receptivity to bacterial adhesion.

The Prevent ADALL study also looked at emollient use but combined this with early introduction of allergenic foods and assessed if this would prevent AD and food allergy. Similarly, it did not find any significant evidence for regular emollient in the prevention of AD; however, early exposure to allergenic foods was found to reduce the prevalence of food allergy at 36 months and was considered a safe strategy to prevent food allergy, with a number needed to treat of 63 [36].

Elimination diets have been discouraged in the prevention of AD and associated atopic disease [37]. In a systemic review and meta-analysis of 10 RCTs, it was found that elimination diets had little effect on AD severity [38]. Indirect evidence from studies on infants with severe AD demonstrated a significant association between peanut elimination and a higher risk of developing peanut allergy and anaphylaxis by age five [39]. Elimination diets also carry a risk of malnutrition and potential care giving burden and hence are not advised.

### 5.2 Personalised medicine

The future of AD treatment is increasingly focused on personalised medicine. This shift is driven by a deeper understanding of the complexity of the disease, and insights from biomarker research, genetic discoveries and microbiome studies.

Research has suggested that the role of certain biomarkers, such as IL-13 levels, may help to predict responses to biological treatment and guide personalised treatment plans.

Genetic research has been pivotal in the understanding of the causes of AD. Genetic discoveries have identified numerous new loci associated with AD, offering potential future treatment targets. In a meta-analysis which looked at over one million individuals, 91 genetic locations were linked to the development of AD, with 32 of these being newly discovered. Another meta-analysis found 77 AD-associated loci, 10 of which were new, with some also linked to inflammatory conditions like inflammatory bowel disease, suggesting shared genetic pathways [40, 41]. This analysis also revealed that certain genetic loci are associated with AD onset in childhood, while others are linked to development later in life [40]. Intriguingly, some of these loci are also connected to other inflammatory conditions like inflammatory bowel disease, suggesting shared genetic pathways [39]. Future research into use of these loci as genetic targets may be pivotal in the discovery of treatment options in the prevention of AD.

Advancements in personalised medicine also include new biologic drugs which target specific cytokines involved in the inflammatory process of AD, such as IL4, IL13, and IL31. Additionally, the use of Janus kinase (JAK) inhibitors, specifically those that inhibit JAK1 and JAK2, has also shown promise in the treatment of AD [42].

AD is characterised by changes in the skin's microbiome, known as dysbiosis. Staphylococcus species, specifically *S. aureus*, has been known to dominate the microbial environment [43, 44]. Research has shown that damaged skin cells release a host protein which inhibits Rnase 7, a protein that normally protects the skin from *S. aureus*. The inhibition leads to increased inflammation and overgrowth of *S. aureus* [42–44]. A meta-analysis confirmed *S. aureus* colonisation in 70% of affected skin and 39% of unaffected skin in AD patients. Targeting the skin microbiome is a promising area for treatment, with narrow-band UVB light therapy shown to improve the microbiome of affected skin in AD patients, reducing *S. aureus* and increasing microbial diversity. Systemic treatments like Dupilumab also have a role in the reversal of skin dysbiosis [44]. Probiotics have also had a role in the skin's microbiome, and this area continues to be a potential research area for AD treatment [45].

## 6. Conclusion

AD is a complex, chronic inflammatory skin condition driven by a dysfunctional epidermal barrier, immune dysregulation, and environmental factors. Family history is an important risk factor. While early and regular introduction of common food allergens in infants has proven effective in preventing food allergies, general emollient use for AD prevention has shown limited direct benefit, with some studies even suggesting an increased risk of skin infections. Dietary elimination for AD is strongly discouraged due to the lack of evidence of improvement and the significant danger of establishing new food allergies, particularly in newborns, as well as potential nutritional inadequacies and carer load.

While RAST and other conventional techniques were essential for detecting IgE antibodies, modern and more sensitive immunoassays have replaced them. Nonetheless, OFC continues to be the most reliable method for identifying food allergies. Particularly in children, OFCs are essential for confirming clinical reactivity, differentiating between sensitisation and true allergy, and evaluating allergy resolution. OFCs avoid dietary restrictions and guide individualised nutritional management.

Treatment for AD is evolving towards a personalised approach. Genetic research has identified numerous new AD-associated loci, opening avenues for genetically targeted interventions and new ways to balance the microbiome. The evolving understanding of AD's pathogenesis, integrated with advancements in the understanding of genetics, biomarkers, and the microbiome promises more effective management and improved outcomes for patients with this atopic condition. It is preferable to include a conclusion(s) section which will summarise the content of the book chapter.

## Conflict of interest

The authors declare no conflict of interest.

## Notes/thanks/other declarations

I would like to express my sincere gratitude to Dr. Nader Elgharably and Miss Samar Shoeir for their invaluable guidance, unwavering support, and dedication to my education. Their tireless efforts have been instrumental in shaping my academic journey and fostering my growth.

My heartfelt thanks also go to Tante Amar for her continuous kindness and unwavering support which is a source of strength and comfort.

## Author details

Noura Elgharably* and Nadir Omar
Croydon University Hospital, London, England

*Address all correspondence to: noura.elgharably4@nhs.net; mohammed.abadie@nhs.net

## References

[1] Bieber T. Atopic dermatitis 2.0: From the clinical phenotype to the molecular taxonomy and stratified medicine. Allergy. 2012;**67**(12):1475-1482. DOI: 10.1111/all.12049

[2] Kim JP et al. Persistence of atopic dermatitis (AD): A systematic review and meta-analysis. Journal of the American Academy of Dermatology. 2016;**75**(4):681-687.e11. DOI: 10.1016/j.jaad.2016.05.028

[3] Weidinger S et al. Atopic dermatitis. Nature Reviews Disease Primers. 2018;**4**(Article 1). DOI: 10.1038/s41572-018-0001-z

[4] Lack G et al. Factors associated with the development of Peanut allergy in childhood. New England Journal of Medicine. 2003;**348**(11):977-985. DOI: 10.1056/nejmoa013536

[5] Justiz Vaillant AA, Modi P, Syed HA, et al. Atopy. In: StatPearls [Internet]. Treasure Island (FL): StatPearls Publishing; 2025. Available from: https://www.ncbi.nlm.nih.gov/books/NBK542187/ [Accessed: June 8, 2025]

[6] Böhme M et al. Family history and risk of atopic dermatitis in children up to 4 years. Clinical and Experimental Allergy. 2003;**33**(9):1226-1231. DOI: 10.1046/j.1365-2222.2003.01749.x

[7] Wollenberg A et al. ETFAD/EADV eczema task force 2020 position paper on diagnosis and treatment of atopic dermatitis in adults and children. Journal of the European Academy of Dermatology and Venereology. 2020;**34**(12):2717-2744. DOI: 10.1111/jdv.16892

[8] Ravn NH et al. How does parental history of atopic disease predict the risk of atopic dermatitis in a child? A systematic review and meta-analysis. Journal of Allergy and Clinical Immunology. 2019;**145**(4):1182-1193. DOI: 10.1016/j.jaci.2019.12.899

[9] Cork MJ et al. Epidermal barrier dysfunction in atopic dermatitis. Journal of Investigative Dermatology. 2009;**129**(8):1892-1908. DOI: 10.1038/jid.2009.133

[10] Kezic S, Jakasa I. Filaggrin and skin barrier function. Current Problems in Dermatology. 2016;**49**:1-7. DOI: 10.1159/000441539

[11] Howell MD et al. Cytokine modulation of atopic dermatitis filaggrin skin expression. Journal of Allergy and Clinical Immunology. 2007;**120**(1):150-155. DOI: 10.1016/j.jaci.2007.04.031

[12] Kishibe M. Physiological and pathological roles of kallikrein-related peptidases in the epidermis. Journal of Dermatological Science. 2019;**95**(2):50-55. DOI: 10.1016/j.jdermsci.2019.06.007

[13] Kim J, Kim BE, Leung DYM. Pathophysiology of atopic dermatitis: Clinical implications. Allergy and Asthma Proceedings. 2019;**40**(2):84-92. DOI: 10.2500/aap.2019.40.4202

[14] Boothe WD, Tarbox JA, Tarbox MB. Atopic dermatitis: Pathophysiology. Advances in Experimental Medicine and Biology. 2024;**1447**:21-35. DOI: 10.1007/978-3-031-54513-9_3

[15] Langan SM, Irvine AD, Weidinger S. Atopic dermatitis. The Lancet. 2020;**396**(10247):345-360. DOI: 10.1016/s0140-6736(20)31286-1

[16] Fox AT et al. Household peanut consumption as a risk factor for the

development of peanut allergy. Journal of Allergy and Clinical Immunology. 2009;**123**(2):417-423. DOI: 10.1016/j.jaci.2008.12.014

[17] Brough HA et al. Peanut allergy: Effect of environmental peanut exposure in children with filaggrin loss-of-function mutations. Journal of Allergy and Clinical Immunology. 2014;**134**(4):867-875.e1. DOI: 10.1016/j.jaci.2014.08.011

[18] Chu DK et al. Atopic dermatitis (eczema) guidelines: 2023 American Academy of allergy, asthma and immunology/American College of Allergy, asthma and immunology joint task force on practice parameters GRADE– And Institute of Medicine–based recommendations. Annals of Allergy, Asthma & Immunology. 2023;**132**(3):274-312. DOI: 10.1016/j.anai.2023.11.009

[19] Elgharably N, Abadie MA. The relationship between atopic dermatitis and food allergy. European Journal of Pharmaceutical Research. 2024;**4**(1):1-4. DOI: 10.24018/ejpharma.2024.4.1.75

[20] Berg T, Bennich H, Johansson SGO. Diagnosis of atopic allergy. International Archives of Allergy and Immunology. 1971;**40**(6):770-778. DOI: 10.1159/000230461

[21] Johansson SGO. Discovery and development of IgE assays. Clinical and Experimental Allergy. 1997;**27**(s1):60-63. DOI: 10.1111/j.1365-2222.1997.tb01828.x

[22] Lis K, Bartuzi Z. Selected technical aspects of molecular allergy diagnostics. Current Issues in Molecular Biology. 2023;**45**(7):5481-5493. DOI: 10.3390/cimb45070347

[23] Schoefer Y et al. Predictivity of allergic sensitization (RAST) for the onset of allergic diseases in adults. Allergy. 2007;**63**(1):81-86. DOI: 10.1111/j.1398-9995.2007.01517.x

[24] Al-Abadie M et al. The role of radioallergosorbent testing (RAST) early in the management of atopic dermatitis in children and adults referred to secondary care in the United Kingdom. International Journal of Clinical and Experimental Dermatology. 2019;**4**(2):1-4. DOI: 10.33140/ijced.04.02.03

[25] Salazar A et al. Allergen-based diagnostic: Novel and old methodologies with new approaches. In: Allergen. InTech; 2017. DOI: 10.5772/intechopen.69276

[26] Negrini AC, Troise C, Voltolini S. ELISA in diagnosis of respiratory allergy. Allergy. 1985;**40**(4):238-241. DOI: 10.1111/j.1398-9995.1985.tb00227.x

[27] Calvani M et al. Oral food challenge. Medicina. 2019;**55**(10):651. DOI: 10.3390/medicina55100651

[28] Sicherer SH. Food allergy: When and how to perform oral food challenges. Pediatric Allergy and Immunology. 1999;**10**(4):226-234. DOI: 10.1034/j.1399-3038.1999.00040.x

[29] Lieberman JA, Sicherer SH. Diagnosis of food allergy: Epicutaneous skin tests, in vitro tests, and oral food challenge. Current Allergy and Asthma Reports. 2010;**11**(1):58-64. DOI: 10.1007/s11882-010-0149-4

[30] Santos AF et al. EAACI guidelines on the diagnosis of IgE-mediated food allergy. Allergy. 2023;**78**(12):3057-3076. DOI: 10.1111/all.15902

[31] Sampson HA et al. AAAAI–EAACI PRACTALL: Standardizing oral food challenges—2024 update. Pediatric Allergy and Immunology. 2024;**35**(11):e14276. DOI: 10.1111/pai.14276

[32] Foong R-X et al. Improving diagnostic accuracy in food allergy. The Journal of Allergy and Clinical Immunology in Practice. 2021;**9**(1):71-80. DOI: 10.1016/j.jaip.2020.09.037

[33] Adkinson NF, Hamilton RG. Clinical history–driven diagnosis of allergic diseases: Utilizing in vitro IgE testing. The Journal of Allergy and Clinical Immunology in Practice. 2015;**3**(6):871-876. DOI: 10.1016/j.jaip.2015.08.002

[34] Hamilton RG, Adkinson NF. Clinical laboratory assessment of IgE-dependent hypersensitivity. Journal of Allergy and Clinical Immunology. 2003;**111**(2):S687-S701. DOI: 10.1067/mai.2003.123

[35] Chalmers JR et al. Daily emollient during infancy for prevention of eczema: The BEEP randomised controlled trial. The Lancet. 2020;**395**(10228):962-972. DOI: 10.1016/s0140-6736(19)32984-8

[36] Skjerven HO et al. Early food intervention and skin emollients to prevent food allergy in young children (PreventADALL): A factorial, multicentre, cluster-randomised trial. The Lancet. 2022;**399**(10344):2398-2411. DOI: 10.1016/s0140-6736(22)00687-0

[37] Oykhman P et al. Dietary elimination for the treatment of atopic dermatitis: A systematic review and meta-analysis. The Journal of Allergy and Clinical Immunology in Practice. 2022;**10**(10):2657-2666.e8. DOI: 10.1016/j.jaip.2022.06.044

[38] Keet C et al. Age and eczema severity, but not family history, are major risk factors for peanut allergy in infancy. Journal of Allergy and Clinical Immunology. 2021;**147**(3):984-991.e5. DOI: 10.1016/j.jaci.2020.11.033

[39] Shi X, Chen Q, Wang F. The bidirectional association between inflammatory bowel disease and atopic dermatitis: A systematic review and meta-analysis. Dermatology. 2020;**236**(6):546-553. DOI: 10.1159/000505290

[40] Budu-Aggrey A, Kilanowski A, Sobczyk MK, et al. European and multi-ancestry genome-wide association meta-analysis of atopic dermatitis highlights importance of systemic immune regulation. Nature Communications. 2023;**14**(1):6172. DOI: 10.1038/s41467-023-41180-2

[41] Fishbein AB et al. Update on atopic dermatitis: Diagnosis, severity assessment, and treatment selection. The Journal of Allergy and Clinical Immunology in Practice. 2019;**8**(1):91-101. DOI: 10.1016/j.jaip.2019.06.044

[42] Rademacher F et al. Inhibition of RNase 7 by RNase inhibitor promotes inflammation and *Staphylococcus aureus* growth: Implications for atopic dermatitis. Allergy. 2024;**79**(6):1573-1583. DOI: 10.1111/all.16125

[43] Kashaf SS et al. Staphylococcal diversity in atopic dermatitis from an individual to a global scale. Cell Host & Microbe. 2023;**31**(4):578-592.e6. DOI: 10.1016/j.chom.2023.03.010

[44] Hülpüsch C et al. Exploring the skin microbiome in atopic dermatitis pathogenesis and disease modification. Journal of Allergy and Clinical Immunology. 2024;**154**(1):31-41. DOI: 10.1016/j.jaci.2024.04.029

[45] Kang S-H et al. Probiotic consumption alleviates atopic dermatitis-related immune responses in association with gut microbial changes: In vitro and mouse model studies. Journal of Functional Foods. 2024;**121**:106428. DOI: 10.1016/j.jff.2024.106428

Chapter 2

# Biological Treatments in Atopic Dermatitis: Current Treatments and Future Directions

*Muhammed Ali Mergen, Tubanur Cetinarslan and Aylin Turel Ermertcan*


## Abstract

Atopic dermatitis (AD) is a chronic and relapsing inflammatory skin disease characterized by intense pruritus, recurrent eczematous lesions and lichenification. It is a heterogeneous disease affecting both children and adults. The treatment choice of moderate-to-severe forms is challenging. Fortunately, systemic treatments can be considered in patients with AD refractory to topical treatments. Numerous biological treatments have been approved to treat AD in case of insufficient disease control with topical therapies and/or significant side effects of conventional systemic therapies. This chapter includes general information about current biological treatment modalities and future directions in AD. The objective is to provide guidance on which patients should be treated with biologics, as well as detailed information on each biological treatment including dupilumab, tralokinumab and lebrikizumab and to report on new developments about investigational biological therapies including nemolizumab, eblasakimab and agents targeting OX40/OX40L (telazorlimab, rocatinlimab and amlitelimab). In this chapter, multicentered randomized studies, systematic reviews, guidelines and clinical trials were used to collect information about biologics. A comprehensive review of current biological therapies that include concurrent use of topical treatments, dosages, tapering, mechanism of action, efficacy, adverse effects, monitoring parameters and contraindications was reported in this chapter. Furthermore, an overview of the literature on promising biological treatments in the future in AD that evaluates the mechanism of action, clinical efficacy, limitations and prospects was reported. Thus, this chapter provides evidence to guide the optimal choice of biological therapy in patients with AD.


**Keywords:** atopic dermatitis, biologics, dupilumab, pediatric, investigational biologics

## 1. Introduction

Atopic dermatitis (AD) is a chronic and relapsing inflammatory skin disease. It has been described as an intense itch and inflammatory eczema in ancient times. Till now, its most prominent feature is still itching [1]. Therefore, it is characterized by intense pruritus, recurrent eczematous lesions and lichenification. AD is one the most common chronic diseases worldwide, affecting one in every five to ten people in developed countries. However, in developing countries, its prevalence is less, yet it is getting higher in time [2, 3]. Although it manifests during the first year of life in most of the cases, it can begin at any age. It is a heterogeneous disease, affecting both children and adults [4–6]. In 70–80% of patients, the disease severity is mild and improves by late childhood. However, the burden of symptoms in children with early-onset with no improvement or patients with adult-onset with moderate-to-severe disease may be profound [1, 6]. It may disrupt the quality of life and sleep of patients, their social activities and occupational and school success [6, 7].

## 2. Pathogenesis of AD and the role of biologics

The main causes that initiate the pathogenesis of AD are thought to be epidermal barrier dysfunction, immune dysregulation, environmental and microbiological factors. These factors trigger inflammation in the skin through various pathways [8, 9]. Epidermal barrier is disrupted due to decreased filaggrin production, protease-antiprotease imbalance, microbial colonization and proinflammatory cytokine release [10–12]. Disruption of the barrier facilitates transcutaneous passage of allergens and microbial agents [12]. These agents cause the release of danger signals (alarmins). Alarmins activate dendritic epidermal cells and type-2 immune cells [8]. After Langerhans cells encounter allergens and pathogens, OX40-Ligand is expressed. The expression of OX40L and the stimulation of alarmins activate antigen-presenting cells (APC), leading to more OX40-Ligand production. Similarly, naive T cells, stimulated by alarmins, express OX40. APC present antigen to naive T cells *via* OX40-OX40-Ligand bridges, enhancing T-cell survival, proliferation and cytotoxicity and cytokine release. Activation of T cells triggers T-cell-mediated immune response [13, 14].

Amlitelimab binds to OX40-Ligand on APC, while rocatinlimab and telazorlimab bind to OX40 on activated T cells, aiming to block the costimulation pathway and modulate persistent inflammation (**Figure 1**) [15–17].

Even though primarily Th-2-mediated immune response is activated, Th1, Th17 and Th22-mediated immune responses are also activated. Activation of nontype 2 pathways causes the release of proinflammatory cytokines such as IFN-gamma, IL-17 and IL-22, thus causing skin inflammation. Activation of type-2 immune response increases expressions of IL-4, IL-5, IL-13 and IL-31 [12]. Thus, B cells are activated and IgE is synthesized. Inflammation is exacerbated through IgE antibodies and degranulation of mast cells, eosinophils and neutrophils. IL-4 and IL-13 downregulate skin barrier proteins and lipids and further increase skin barrier dysfunction [12, 18, 19]. While IL-4 and IL-13 indirectly, IL-31 directly activate sensory neurons, causing pruritus and initiating the itch-scratch cycle [20, 21]. As a result, the skin barrier deteriorates and lichenification occurs due to keratinocyte proliferation and epidermal thickening.

Dupilumab blocks IL-4 and IL-13 signaling by binding to IL-4Rα [22]. Tralokinumab and lebrikizumab inhibit the activation of IL-4R-alpha/IL13R1-alpha receptor by binding to IL-13 [23, 24]. Eblasakimab inhibits IL-4/IL-13 signaling by

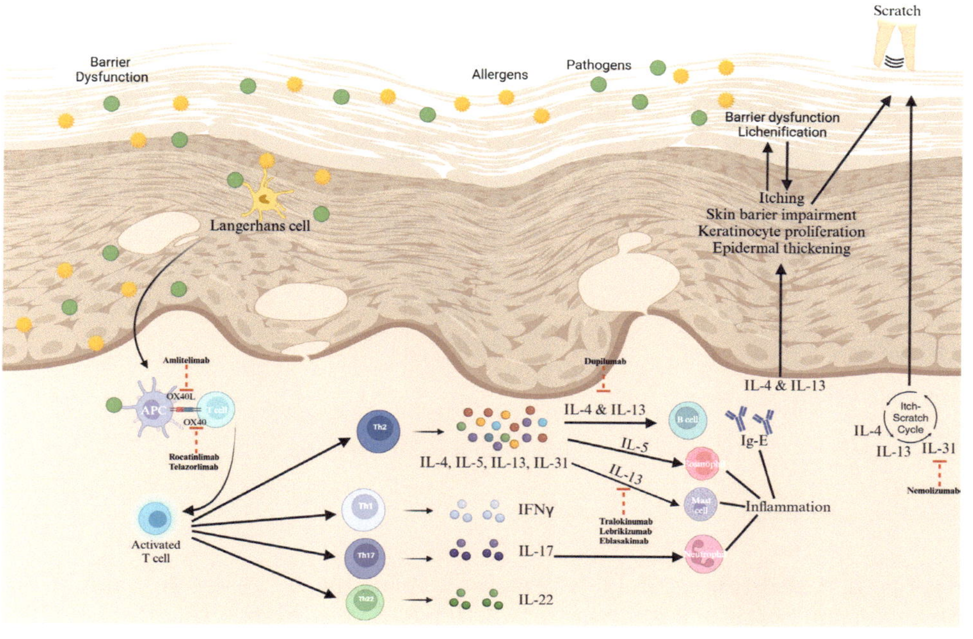


**Figure 1.**
*Pathogenesis of AD and The Role of Biologics.*

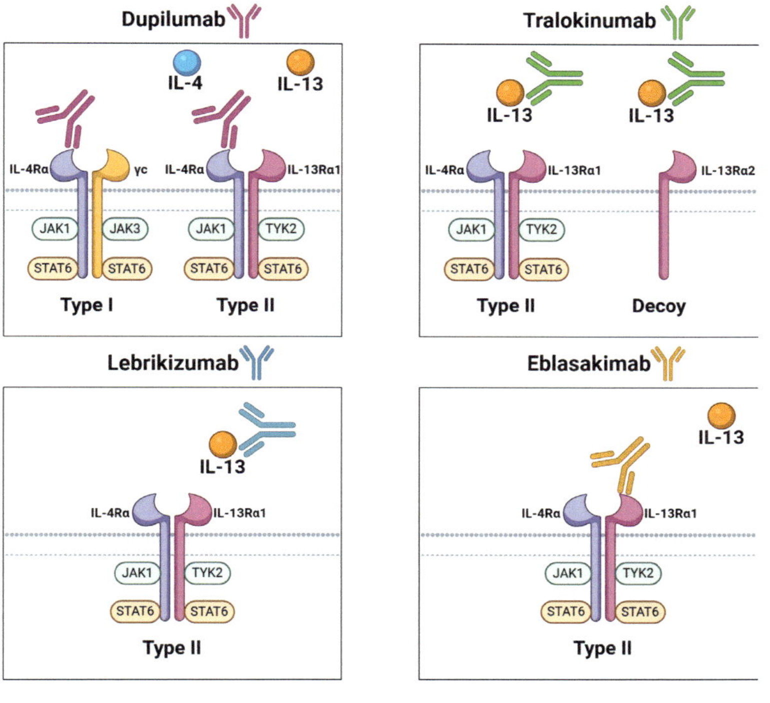


**Figure 2.**
*Biologics and their mechanism of IL-4 and IL-13 inhibition.*

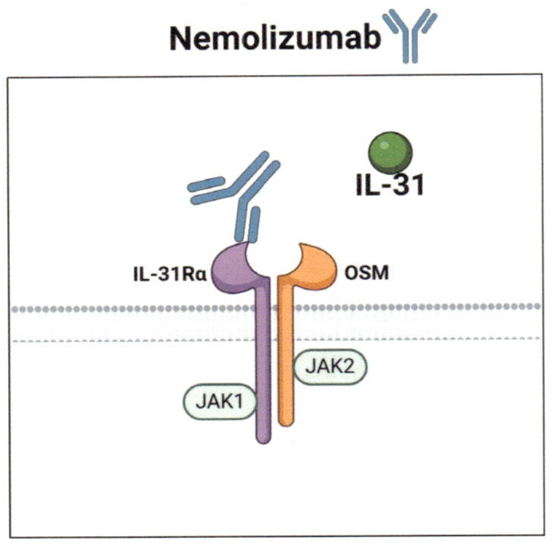


**Figure 3.**
*Nemolizumab and its mechanism of IL-31 inhibition.*

blocking IL-13Rα1 (**Figure 2**) [25]. Nemolizumab inhibits IL-31 signaling and, thus, the nonhistaminergic itch pathway by targeting IL-31R-α (**Figure 3**) [26].

## 3. Evaluation of disease severity and selection of biological therapy

In assessing the severity of AD, morphology and extent of rash (redness, swelling, oozing/crusting, scratch, skin thickening and dryness), effects of symptoms such as itching or pain on daily activities and sleep quality, frequency of flares and chronicity are taken into consideration [27]. In addition, unresolved itching and lichenification may be signs of a more severe clinical picture than might be expected due to the lack of visible erythema in darkly pigmented skin. Scoring AD (SCORAD), Eczema Area and Severity Index (EASI), Investigator Global Assessment (IGA) and Peak Pruritus-Numerical rating scale (PP-NRS) are widely used severity assessment methods in guidelines, clinical studies and randomized controlled trials [27–30]. In European guideline on AD, candidates for systemic treatment had been defined as patients with SCORAD more than 50, or patients with no response to adequate topical treatments, or patients whose daily activities are negatively affected despite adequate treatment. Azathioprine (AZA), methotrexate (MTX), cyclosporine (CyA), dupilumab, tralokinumab, upadacitinib and baricitinib were recommended to systemic treatment candidates with a personalized plan considering factors such as age of the patients, side effects of the treatments, onset of effect of the treatment and effectiveness of the treatment [31]. In the update of the American Academy of Dermatology (AAD)'s 2024 recommendations, dupilumab, tralokinumab, upadacitinib, abrocitinib and baricitinib had been strongly recommended while systemic conventional therapies and phototherapy had been conditionally recommended [32].

## 4. Biological agents

In this section, biological agents that are approved (dupilumab, tralokinumab, lebrikizumab and nemolizumab) and those in ongoing studies (eblasakimab, amlitelimab, rocatinlimab and telazorlimab) for patients with moderate-to-severe AD, unresponsive to topical treatments are discussed.

### 4.1 Dupilumab

Dupilumab binds to IL-4Rα subunit of IL-4Rα/γc receptor complex and IL-4Rα/IL-13Rα1 receptor complex. Thus, it interferes with IL-4 and IL-13 signaling elicited *via* type 1 and type 2 receptors (**Figure 2**) [22, 33]. Receptor blockade results in downregulation of inflammatory mediators and epidermal proliferation markers and upregulation of genes involved in skin barrier function.

Dupilumab was approved by the Food and Drug Administration (FDA) in June 2022 and by the European Medicines Agency (EMA) in March 2023 for adults and children aged 6 months or older with moderate-to-severe AD, unresponsive to adequate topical treatments [34, 35].

#### *4.1.1 Efficacy*

In SOLO-1 and SOLO-2 studies conducted in adults; the percentages of patients reaching IGA 0/1, EASI-50, EASI-75 and EASI-90 responses in dupilumab monotherapy at week 16 were significantly higher than those with placebo [36]. The percentages of patients reaching EASI-75 response were 51 and 44% in the dupilumab groups and 14% and 11% in the placebo groups, respectively. Similarly, a significantly greater decrease in the initial pruritus score was found in the dupilumab groups compared to placebo. Improvement in pruritus in the dupilumab groups began at day 2 in adults and day 5 in adolescents. This rapid response was thought to be due to the prevention of pruritus induction due to IL-4R-alpha inhibition. Additionally, significant improvements in quality of life, anxiety and depression scores were observed in the dupilumab groups at week 16 compared to placebo [36].

Similar to SOLO-1 and SOLO-2, in the CHRONOS study conducted in adults, the primary and secondary endpoints were significantly reached in the dupilumab and topical corticosteroid (TCS) combination compared to placebo at week 16 [36]. The efficacy continued in the majority of patients receiving dupilumab until week 52. The percentage of patients who maintained their EASI-75 response was 65% in the dupilumab group, while it was 21% in placebo group [36].

In the LIBERTY AD CHRONOS study, the percentages of patients who maintained their EASI response at week 52 in the dupilumab every 2 weeks (q2w) and once weekly (qw) groups were examined [37]. In the dupilumab groups, 79–70% of patients maintained their EASI-50 response, 65–64% of patients maintained their EASI-75 response and 51–51% of patients maintained their EASI-90 response, respectively, which were significantly higher than those in placebo [37].

In the AD-1526 study conducted in adolescents, the percentages of patients achieving IGA 0/1 response and EASI-75 response were found to be significantly higher in dupilumab groups compared to placebo. At week 16, the percentage of patients achieving an EASI-50 response was 61% and the percentage of patients achieving an EASI-75 response was 41% [38].

In a study conducted on children aged 6 months to 6 years, efficacy and safety were investigated in the combination of dupilumab and TCS. The percentage of those reaching IGA 0/1 response at week 16 (28–4%) was found to be significantly higher than placebo [39].

#### 4.1.2 Administration and dosage

In children, adolescents and adults over 60 kg, it is recommended to initially administer 600 mg subcutaneous (sc) injection followed by 300 mg sc injection every 2 weeks. In adolescents under 60 kg, it is recommended to initially administer 400 mg sc injection followed by 200 mg injection every 2 weeks. In children under 60 kg, injections should be made with special dose adjustments according to weight [34].

#### 4.1.3 Drug interactions

Dupilumab is not expected to be metabolized by hepatic enzymes or renal elimination [34, 35]. Clinically important interactions between dupilumab and inhibitors, inducers or substrates of CYP1A2, CYP3A, CYPC19, CYP2D6 or CYP2C9 enzymes are not expected and no dose adjustment is required. However, dupilumab may diminish the therapeutic effect of Fc Receptor-Binding Agents and may enhance the adverse/toxic effect of live vaccines [34, 35]. Age-appropriate vaccinations should be done according to current immunization guidelines prior to dupilumab therapy. However, live vaccines should not be given right before and during the treatment with dupilumab [34, 35].

#### 4.1.4 Monitoring parameters

In studies conducted in adults, adolescents and children, no laboratory abnormalities other than transient eosinophilia were detected in patients receiving dupilumab. Thus, screening and routine laboratory monitoring was not considered necessary [40–42].

#### 4.1.5 Adverse events

Dupilumab-associated adverse events were mostly injection site reactions, dupilumab-associated ocular surface disease (DAOSD), nasopharyngitis, facial erythema and transient eosinophilia and less frequently psoriasiform dermatitis, seronegative arthritis/enthesitis and herpes infections [43]. Serious/opportunistic infections were similar with placebo and non-herpetic skin infection percentages were lower than placebo. The likely mechanism is inhibition of IL-4 and IL-13 signaling, which leads to the itch-scratch cycle and downregulation of skin barrier proteins and lipids. Therefore, dupilumab is thought to be an immunomodulator rather than an immunosuppressant [43].

DAOSD such as conjunctivitis, blepharitis, keratitis, dry eye and severe blepharoconjunctivitis were observed in 11–26% of cases [44–47]. Ocular side effects mostly begin two weeks to four months after the first injection. Most cases were mild to moderate in severity [44]. No ocular side effects had been observed when dupilumab was used for asthma or other diseases [47]. Therefore, it is thought that an underlying subclinical ocular disease has emerged. Severe AD and a history of allergic conjunctivitis are thought to be the risk factors for developing ocular side effects after dupilumab injections [47]. In the prevention and treatment of ocular side effects, lubricants and preservative-free eye drops can be used. Anti-inflammatory eye drops or ointments containing corticosteroids, calcineurin inhibitors or cyclosporine can also be used in the treatment of mild to moderate conjunctivitis. If ocular side effects persists or is severe, patients should be referred to an ophtalmologist [44–47].

Dupilumab-associated facial erythema is defined as an exacerbation or new onset of head and neck dermatitis and occurs in 4–10% of adults and up to 29% of adolescents [48]. It usually begins approximately two months after the first injection. Although the pathogenesis is unclear, subclinical psoriasis, TCS deprivation and demodex proliferation are possible mechanisms. TCS, topical antifungal medications and topical ivermectin may be used for treatment [48].

According to VigiBASE (Who Global ICSR database), the musculoskeletal system is the third most affected system. Seronegative artritis/enthesitis usually occurs in the first few months. Th17 axis activation after blockade of Th2 immune response is blamed. Paradoxical Th17 emergence causes arthritis and uveitis. They are mostly mild and conservative treatment is sufficient [49].

#### *4.1.6 Contraindications*

A history of hypersensitivity reaction to dupilumab or any component of the formulation. No dosage adjustment is required for liver/kidney impairment [35].

#### *4.1.7 Special considerations: Pregnancy, lactation and comorbidities*

There is no direct or indirect fetal toxicity in animal studies [35]. It has no effect on fertility [34]. A case report of dupilumab treatment in severe AD during pregnancy showed no adverse maternal or fetal outcomes [50]. However, there is insufficient data before, during and after pregnancy [35]. Dupilumab is excreted in breastmilk but it is not known whether it is absorbed by oral intake [34]. In a consensus report in Northern Europe, CyA was the first choice systemic treatment before conception, during and after pregnancy. No consensus was reached on the use of dupilumab as a second option before and during pregnancy [50, 51]. Thus, dupilumab should be given during and after pregnancy only if benefits to mother and/or fetus or child outweigh any potential risk to the fetus or child [34].

The European guideline has reported that dupilumab treatment may be beneficial for type 2 comorbidities like asthma, eosinophilic esophagitis and allergic conjunctivitis [31]. Therefore, in pediatric patients with moderate-to-severe AD, dupilumab can be considered as a good option in the presence of atopic comorbidity, high serum total IgE level and family history of atopy [52].

#### *4.1.8 Comparison with other systemic treatment modalities*

Heads-Up study compared the efficacy and safety of 30 mg oral upadacitinib once daily with 300 mg sc dupilumab administration every other week for 16 weeks in 673 patients with moderate-to-severe AD [53]. At week 16, 72.4% of patients receiving upadacitinib and 62.62% of patients receiving dupilumab achieved an EASI75 response. Upadacitinib (30 mg/day) was found to be superior in achieving EASI 90 and EASI 100 responses and in improving pruritus. The rates of serious infections, eczema herpeticum, herpes zoster and laboratory-related adverse events were higher in patients receiving upadacitinib. In contrast, the rates of conjunctivitis and injection site reactions were higher in patients receiving dupilumab [53].

In a study conducted in 838 patients with AD who were unresponsive to topical treatments or required systemic treatment, the efficacy of oral abrocitinib 200 mg or 100 mg once daily was compared with dupilumab 300 mg subcutaneously administration every other week [54]. The percentages of patients who achieved IGA 0/1 response at week 12 were 48.4% in the group receiving 200 mg abrocitinib, 36.6% in the group receiving 100 mg abrocitinib, 36.5% in the group receiving dupilumab and 14% in the placebo group. The percentages of patients achieving EASI-75 response were observed in 70.3, 58.7, 58.1 and 27.1%, respectively. At week 16, no significant difference was observed in important secondary endpoints between the abrocitinib 200 mg/day or 100 mg/day groups and dupilumab group [54].

A meta-analysis of 60 RCTs with more than 16,000 participants compared all systemic therapies in the treatment of AD [55]. The outcomes were EASI, Patient-Oriented Eczema Measure (POEM), Dermatology Life Quality Index (DLQI) and P-NRS. There was a consistent pattern among the outcomes. Dupilumab, abrocitinib, baricitinib, tralokinumab and upadacitinib were associated with improved index scores in adults with moderate-to-severe AD treated for up to 16 weeks [55]. Abrocitinib 200 mg/day and upadacitinib 30 mg/day had higher index scores than dupilumab. Upadacitinib 15 mg/day had similar index scores with dupilumab. Abrocitinib 100 mg/day, baricitinib 2–4 mg/day and systemic conventional therapies had lower index scores than dupilumab [55].

### 4.2 Tralokinumab

Tralokinumab is a fully human IgG4 binding to IL-13. It prevents IL-4Rα/IL-13Rα1 heterodimer receptor complex formation and IL-13Rα2 activation. Thus, it interferes with IL-13 signaling elicited *via* inhibition of only type 2 receptor complex formation (**Figure 2**) [23, 33].

Tralokinumab was approved by the FDA in December 2022 and by the EMA in June 2021 for adult and adolescents aged 12 years or older with moderate-to-severe AD, unresponsive to adequate topical treatments [56, 57].

#### *4.2.1 Efficacy*

In ECZTRA 1 and ECZTRA 2 studies, a total of 1596 patients with AD were administered 300 mg tralokinumab or placebo subcutaneously every other week for 16 weeks [58]. At week 16, the percentages of patients achieving IGA 0/1 response were 16 and 22% in the tralokinumab groups, while they were 7 and 11% in the placebo groups. Similarly, the percentages of patients achieving EASI-75 response were 25 and 33% in the tralokinumab groups, while they were 13 and 11% in the placebo groups, respectively [58]. Tralokinumab was found to be significantly higher than placebo in achieving IGA 0/1 and EASI-75 responses, reducing pruritus and SCORAD baseline scores and improving quality of life at week 16. The percentage of patients maintaining IGA 0/1 response at week 52 was 39% in ECZTRA 1, 45% in ECZTRA 2, and significantly higher than placebo. The percentage of patients maintaining EASI-75 response at week 52 was 49% in ECZTRA 1, 51% in ECZTRA 2, and significantly higher than placebo [58]. A significant proportion of tralokinumab responders at week 16 maintained their response at week 52 with continued treatment [58].

In the ECZTRA 3 study, 300 mg tralokinumab every other week injection and TCS combination were compared with placebo and TCS combination group [59]. The percentage of patients achieving EASI-75 response at week 16 was 56% in tralokinumab-TCS combination and 35% in placebo-TCS combination group. Tralokinumab-TCS combination was significantly higher than placebo-TCS combination in achieving EASI-75 response, reducing pruritus and SCORAD baseline scores and improving quality of life at week 16 [59]. Of the responders at week 16, 89.6 and 92.5% of those treated every 2 weeks (q2w) and 77.6 and 90.8% of those treated every 4 weeks (q4w) maintained IGA 0/1 and EASI 75 responses at week 32, respectively [59].

In ECZTRA-6 study conducted in 289 patients aged 12–17 years with moderate-to-severe AD, tralokinumab was found to be more effective than placebo in achieving IGA 0/1 and EASI-75 responses at week 16 [60].

#### *4.2.2 Administration and dosage*

In adults and adolescents aged 12 years or more, it is recommended to initially administer 600 mg sc injection followed by 300 mg sc injection every other week [56, 57].

#### *4.2.3 Drug interactions*

Tralokinumab is not expected to be metabolized by hepatic enzymes or renal elimination [56]. Clinically important interactions between tralokinumab and inhibitors, inducers or substrates of CYP1A2, CYP2C9, CYP2D6, CYP2C19 and CYP3A enzymes are not expected and no dose adjustment is required [57]. EMA states that there are no adverse interactions between non-live vaccines and tralokinumab [57]. However, tralokinumab may diminish the therapeutic effect of Fc Receptor-Binding Agents and may enhance the adverse/toxic effect of live vaccines [56, 57]. Age-appropriate vaccinations should be done by current immunization guidelines prior to tralokinumab therapy. Non-live vaccines may be given concurrently with tralokinumab therapy. However, live and live-attenuated vaccines should not be given during the treatment with tralokinumab [57].

#### *4.2.4 Monitoring parameters*

In studies conducted in adults and adolescents aged 12 years or more, no laboratory abnormalities were detected in patients receiving tralokinumab through 52 weeks of follow-up [61, 62]. Thus, screening and routine laboratory monitoring was not considered necessary [61, 62].

#### *4.2.5 Adverse events*

Tralokinumab-associated adverse events were mostly upper respiratory tract infections (16%), allergic conjunctivitis (5%) and injection site reactions (3%) [58, 61]. It was determined that the rate of ocular side effects was lower in patients receiving tralokinumab than in patients receiving dupilumab. The possible mechanism for the lower rate of ocular side effects was thought to be that tralokinumab does not block type 1 receptors [58, 63]. Additionally, a reduction in eczema herpeticum and skin infections requiring systemic treatment was observed in patients receiving tralokinumab compared to placebo [58].

#### *4.2.6 Contraindications*

A history of hypersensitivity reaction to tralokinumab or any component of the formulation. No dosage adjustment is required for liver/kidney impairment [56, 57].

#### *4.2.7 Pregnancy and lactation*

Pregnancy and lactation category is unknown due to insufficient data in women of childbearing potential. There is no direct or indirect fetal toxicity in animal studies [64].

#### *4.2.8 Comparison with other systemic treatment modalities*

A meta-analysis of 60 RCTs with more than 16,579 participants compared all systemic therapies in the treatment of AD [55]. The outcomes were EASI, POEM, DLQI and P-NRS. There was a consistent pattern among the outcomes. Dupilumab, abrocitinib, baricitinib, tralokinumab and upadacitinib were associated with improved index scores in adults with moderate-to-severe AD treated for up to 16 weeks [55]. Abrocitinib 200 mg/day, upadacitinib 30 mg/day or 15 mg/day and dupilumab 600 mg then 300 mg every other week had higher index scores than tralokinumab [55].

### 4.3 Lebrikizumab

Lebrikizumab is a fully human IgG4 binding to IL-13. It prevents IL-4Rα/IL-13Rα1 heterodimer receptor complex formation. Thus, it interferes with IL-13 signaling elicited *via* inhibition of just type 2 receptor complex formation (**Figure 2**) [24, 33].

Lebrikizumab was approved by the FDA in September 2024 and by the EMA in November 2023 for adult and adolescents aged 12 years or older with a body weight of at least 40 kg who are candidates for systemic treatment in AD [65, 66].

#### *4.3.1 Efficacy*

In ADvocate 1 and 2 studies conducted in 851 patients with moderate-to-severe AD, treatment responses of lebrikizumab and placebo were compared [67]. At week 16, the percentage of patients who achieved IGA 0/1 response was found to be significantly higher in lebrikizumab groups (43.1 and 33.2%) than in placebo groups (12.7 and 10.8%), respectively. Likewise, the percentages of patients achieving EASI-75 response were 59% and 52% in the lebrikizumab groups, while they were 18 and 6% in the placebo groups, respectively [67]. Additionally, significant improvements in sleep quality and pruritus were observed in lebrikizumab groups compared to placebo [67].

In ADhere study conducted in 211 patients with moderate-to-severe AD, treatment responses of lebrikizumab+TCS combination and placebo+TCS combination were compared [68]. At week 16, the percentage of patients who achieved IGA 0/1 response was found to be significantly higher in lebrikizumab+TCS combination (41%) than in placebo+TCS combination (22%) [68]. The percentages of patients achieving EASI-75 response were 69% in the lebrikizumab+TCs combination, while they were 42% in placebo+TCS combination. Also, significant improvements in quality of life and pruritus were observed in lebrikizumab compared to placebo [68].

A 52-week extension study of the ADvocate1 and ADvocate2 trials investigated the percentage of patients who achieved IGA 0/1 and EASI-75 response at week 16 and maintained at week 52 [69]. 71.2% of patients receiving 250 mg lebrikizumab every other week, 76.9% of patients receiving 250 mg lebrikizumab every four weeks and 47.9% of patients receiving placebo maintained IGA 0/1 score through week 52 [69]. Similarly, 78.4% of patients receiving 250 mg lebrikizumab every other week, 81.7% of patients receiving 250 mg lebrikizumab every four weeks and 66.4% of patients receiving placebo maintained their EASI-75 response through week 52 [69].

In a randomized controlled trial, 16 patients who had not previously benefited from dupilumab treatment were randomized to receive lebrikizumab [24]. At week 16, five of the twelve patients who received lebrikizumab had an EASI-75 response and four had an IGA 0/1 response, while no response was observed in the placebo group [24].

#### *4.3.2 Administration and dosage*

In adult and adolescents aged 12 years or more, it is recommended to initially and at week 2 administer 500 mg sc injection followed by 250 mg sc injection every other week until 16 weeks or later, when adequate clinical response is achieved. The maintenance dose is 250 mg sc injection in every 4 weeks [65, 66].

#### *4.3.3 Drug interactions*

There is no study performed about the safety and efficacy of concurrent use of lebrikizumab and live/live-attenuated vaccines and lebrikizumab and other drug interactions [65, 66]. Thus, live and live-attenuated vaccines should not be given concurrently with lebrikizumab [65, 66]. Lebrikizumab is not expected to be metabolized by hepatic enzymes or renal elimination. As lebrikizumab is a monoclonal antibody, its pharmacokinetic interaction profile is expected to be like dupilumab and tralokinumab [65, 66].

#### *4.3.4 Monitoring parameters*

In studies conducted in adults and adolescents aged 12 years or more, no laboratory abnormalities were detected in patients receiving lebrikizumab through 52 weeks of follow-up. Thus, screening and routine laboratory monitoring was not considered necessary [60, 67–69].

#### *4.3.5 Adverse events*

Lebrikizumab-associated adverse events were mostly conjunctivitis (5–10%), injection site reactions (3%), herpes infections (1%), hypertension and transient eosinophilia [60, 67–69]. Since lebrikizumab, like tralokinumab, does not block type 1 receptors, it was determined that the rate of ocular side effects was lower in patients receiving lebrikizumab than in patients receiving dupilumab [60, 67–69]. Most treatment-emergent adverse events (TEAEs) were nonserious, mild or moderate in intensity and did not lead to study discontinuation [60, 67–69].

#### *4.3.6 Contraindications*

A history of hypersensitivity reaction to lebrikizumab or any component of the formulation. No dosage adjustment is required for liver/kidney impairment [65, 66].

*4.3.7 Pregnancy and lactation*

Pregnancy and lactation category is unknown due to insufficient data in women of childbearing potential. There is no direct or indirect fetal toxicity in animal studies [65, 66].

**4.4 Nemolizumab**

Nemolizumab blocks IL-31R-alpha, thus inhibiting IL-31 signaling and the nonhistaminergic itch pathway (**Figure 3**) [26]. An itch cytokine, IL-31 expression was associated with inflammation, epidermal disruption and itch pathways. In a study examining IL-31 expression in AD and psoriasis patients, IL-31 expression in the lesional skin of patients diagnosed with AD was found to be higher than in the lesional skin of patients diagnosed with psoriasis, in the nonlesional skin of patients diagnosed with AD and psoriasis and in normal individuals [70]. Therefore, it is thought that molecules targeting IL-31 are promising in diseases where itch is an important symptom, such as AD and prurigo. In several studies, nemolizumab was found to be successful in controlling pruritus in patients with AD [21, 70, 71].

Nemolizumab was approved by the FDA in December 2024 for adults and adolescents aged 12 years or older with moderate-to-severe AD, unresponsive to adequate topical treatments. Although evaluations by the EMA are ongoing, its approval of nemolizumab for the same indication seems likely [72].

*4.4.1 Efficacy*

ARCADIA 1–2 studies compared nemolizumab combined with TCS/topical calcineurin inhibitors (TCI) with placebo in 1728 patients aged 12 years and older with moderate-to-severe AD [73]. At week 16, the percentage of patients with IGA 0/1 response was 36% in ARCADIA-1 and 38% in ARCADIA-2, which was higher than placebo [73]. The percentage of patients with EASI-75 response was 44% in ARCADIA-1 and 42% in ARCADIA-2, which was higher than placebo. Similarly, nemolizumab was more effective than placebo in reducing itch and clearing lesions in the subgroup of patients with severe pruritus [73]. Patients who achieved IGA 0/1 and EASI-75 responses with a combination of nemolizumab and TCS/TCI at week 16 were re-randomized and given nemolizumab once a month or once every other month. At week 48, the percentage of patients who maintained their IGA 0/1 response was 63% in the once-monthly group and 64% in those who received it every 2 months. Similarly, 75% of those who received it once a month maintained their EASI-75 response, while 77% of those who received it once every 2 months maintained their EASI-75 response [73].

In a phase 3 double-blind trial, nemolizumab and medium potency TCS/TCI combination was compared with placebo and TCS/TCI combination in patients with moderate-to-severe pruritus and AD [74]. In this trial, lower potency TCS and emollients were allowed. When investigator noted worsening of AD, higher-potency TCS were allowed as rescue therapy and reported as AD worsening. However, there was no consistent definition term for AD worsening. It was accepted after investigators discretion [74]. At week 16, a significant reduction in pruritus was observed in nemolizumab group compared to placebo [74].

In a phase 3 long-term study, nemolizumab and TCS/TCI combination was compared with placebo and TCS/TCI combination in adolescents with moderate-to-severe AD [75]. A significant improvement in EASI, signs of AD, sleep and quality of life and reduction in pruritus was observed in nemolizumab and TCS/TCI combination compared to placebo. Those who received nemolizumab 60 mg/q4w with TCS/TCI maintained responses in pruritus, AD symptoms and quality of life for up to 68 weeks [75].

#### *4.4.2 Administration and dosage*

In adults and adolescents aged 12 years or more, it is recommended to initially administer 60 mg sc injection followed by 30 mg sc injection every month until 16 weeks or later, when adequate clinical response is achieved. The maintenance dose is 30 mg sc injection every 8 weeks [72].

#### *4.4.3 Drug interactions*

Nemolizumab may decrease the serum concentration of CYP substrates and may diminish the therapeutic effect of Fc Receptor-Binding Agents [72]. Nemolizumab may either enhance the adverse/toxic effect or diminish the therapeutic effect of live vaccines. Thus, live and live-attenuated vaccines should not be given concurrently with nemolizumab [72].

#### *4.4.4 Monitoring parameters*

In phase-3 RCT, there were no laboratory abnormalities ledding to discontinuation of nemolizumab treatment [73]. Thus, screening and routine laboratory monitoring was not considered necessary [31].

#### *4.4.5 Adverse events*

Nemolizumab-associated adverse events were mostly headache, arthralgia, urticaria, myalgia, injection site reactions, nasopharyngitis and increased creatinine phoshokinase [73]. TEAEs were generally mild or moderate in severity [31, 73]. In ARCADIA 1 and ARCADIA 2 studies, nemolizumab-related adverse events included worsening of AD (12 and 7% in nemolizumab groups, 11 and 6% in placebo groups) and newly diagnosed asthma or worsening of asthma (5 and 2% in nemolizumab groups, 4 and 3% in placebo groups). Since this was a contradictory situation, the authors explained it as follows [73]. The percentages had been considered high due to the fact that a definition of 'worsening AD' was not used. In these trials, the need for rescue therapy was found to be higher in the placebo group (see: Efficacy (4.4.1)). Since there was a consistent definition for worsening AD in previous phase-2 studies, the rate of worsening AD was higher in placebo than in nemolizumab. A meta-analysis of 688,927 patients found the prevalence of asthma in moderate-to-severe AD patients to be 25%. Similarly, the prevalence was found to be 30% in these trials [73]. According to Center for Disease Control and Prevention (data for year 2021), approximately 40% of patients with asthma are expected to have one or more attacks per year [73]. Therefore, the data on worsening asthma had been considered to reflect normal. Based on this prevalence, the observed incidences of worsening asthma had thought not to constitute evidence of a safety concern [73].

#### *4.4.6 Contraindications*

A history of hypersensitivity reaction to nemolizumab or any component of the formulation. No dosage adjustment is required in liver/kidney impairment [72].

#### *4.4.7 Pregnancy and lactation*

Pregnancy and lactation category is unknown due to insufficient data in women of childbearing potential. There is no direct or indirect fetal toxicity in animal studies [72].

### 4.5 Eblasakimab

Eblasakimab binds to IL-13Rα1 subunit of IL-4Rα/IL-13Rα1 receptor complex. Thus, it interferes with IL-4 and IL-13 signaling elicited *via* inhibition of just type 2 receptor complex formation (**Figure 2**) [25, 33].

Eblasakimab is in early trials for the treatment of AD. A phase 1b, multipl-ascending dose study and a randomized double-blind placebo-controlled phase 2b study in adults has been completed [25, 76, 77].

#### *4.5.1 Efficacy and safety profile*

In a double-blind, multipl-ascending dose, phase 1b study, eblasakimab showed significant improvements compared to placebo in EASI percent change from baseline (%CFBL), proportion of patients achieving EASI50 and EASI75 and PP-NRS %CFBL at week 8 [76]. The decrease in EASI score at the end of week 8 was significantly greater in the group receiving 600 mg eblasakimab weekly compared to placebo. Eblasakimab associated TEAE were mostly injection site reactions, allergic conjunctivitis, headache, rhinorrhea and lethargy. Injection site reactions were detected in 26% of patients and were mild to moderate in severity and transient [76]. Additionally, They did not lead to discontinuation of therapy. Eventhough allergic conjunctivitis were detected higher in eblasakimab groups than in placebo, rates were expected to be similar to lebrikizumab and tralokinumab and lower than dupilumab [76].

In another double-blind, multiple ascending dose, phase 1b study, eblasakimab reduced atopy-associated serum biomarkers such as thymus and activation-regulated chemokine (TARC), total IgE and lactate dehydrogenase in the 400 mg and 600 mg groups at week 8 [25]. Reduction in serum biomarkers associated with AD was thought to be supportive of the significant clinical improvements in EASI, IGA and pruritus scores. These results were consistent with results for dupilumab [25].

In phase-2b TREK-AD trial, the decrease in baseline EASI score at the end of week 16 was significantly greater in the group receiving 600 mg eblasakimab monthly compared to placebo [77]. Most common side effects were conjunctivitis (5.2%) and injection site reactions (4.7%). Eblasakimab demonstrated promising efficacy and safety profile also in this trial [77].

### 4.6 Rocatinlimab

Rocatinlimab binds to OX40 on activated T cells, aiming to block the costimulation pathway and modulate persistent inflammation [16]. Rocatinlimab is in early trials for the treatment of AD. Randomized double-blind placebo-controlled phase 2b studies in adults have been completed [78].

#### *4.6.1 Efficacy and safety profile*

In a multicentre, double-blind, placebo-controlled phase 2b study, rocatinlimab 150 mg or 600 mg every month, 300 mg or 600 mg every other week or placebo were compared up to week 18 [78]. Patients were treated 18 weeks and followed-up 20 weeks more. At week 16, a significant decrease in baseline EASI and IGA scores was observed in the rocatinlimab 300 mg every 2 weeks group compared to placebo. 70% of patients who achieved an EASI-75 response with rocatinlimab treatment maintained their response for up to 20 weeks after treatment discontinuation due to inhibition of Th2 activation and clonal expansion [79]. Since maximum efficacy of dupilumab and upadacitinib was generally observed at week 16 [78, 80], progressive efficacy in rocatinlimab treatment is promising [79]. In the SOLO-CONTINUE study, 30% of patients who achieved an EASI-75 response with dupilumab maintained their response at week 36 after switching to placebo [78]. In the JADE REGIMEN study, 78% of patients who responded to abrocitinib experienced an AD flare after switching to a placebo [81]. The long off-treatment response duration of rocatinlimab differs from current AD treatments [78–81].

Rocatinlimab-associated adverse events were mostly fever, chills, aphthous ulcers and nausea [78]. Since fever and chills mostly occurred after the first injection, they had been considered as injection site reactions. There was no clinically significant change in laboratory parameters, vital signs or electrocardiogram findings in the study [78].

### 4.7 Telazorlimab

Telazorlimab binds to OX40 on activated T cells, aiming to block the costimulation pathway and modulate persistent inflammation [17]. Telazorlimab is in early trials for the treatment of AD. Randomized double-blind placebo-controlled phase 2 studies in adults have been completed [82].

#### *4.7.1 Efficacy and safety profile*

In a placebo-controlled phase 2 study, the efficacy and safety profile of telazorlimab were investigated [82]. At day 71, patients achieving 50% or greater EASI responses was greater with telazorlimab (77%) than placebo (37,5%). Telazorlimab induced reductions in Th1, Th2 and Th17/22 mRNA expression in lesional skin [82]. These reductions persisted 42 days after drug withdrawal. Telazorlimab associated adverse events were mostly headache and at similar rates to placebo. There was no clinically significant change in laboratory values, vital signs or ECG findings in the study [82]. Like rocatinlimab, its progressive efficacy and off-treatment response duration are promising and different from current therapy modalities.

### 4.8 Amlitelimab

Amlitelimab binds to OX40-Ligand on APC, aiming to block the costimulation pathway and modulate persistent inflammation [15, 16]. Amlitelimab is in early trials for the treatment of AD. Randomized double-blind placebo-controlled phase 2 studies in adults have been completed [15].

#### *4.8.1 Efficacy and safety profile*

In a placebo-controlled phase 2 study, similar to rocatinlimab and telazorlimab, amlitelimab demonstrated significant changes compared to placebo in both primary and secondary endpoints at week 16 [15]. Responses were maintained for 24 weeks after treatment discontinuation in patients who achieved an EASI response, an IGA 0/1 response and an improvement in P-NRS score $\geq$ 4 [15].

## 5. Conclusions

AD is chronic and relapsing inflammatory skin disease characterized by intense pruritus, recurrent eczematous lesions and lichenification. The treatment choice of moderate-to-severe forms is challenging. Fortunately, there are several systemic treatment options in patients with AD refractory to adequate topical therapies. An important part of these systemic treatment options is biological treatment. Among FDA and/or EMA-approved treatments, dupilumab is associated with higher index scores in primary and secondary outcome measures compared to IL-13 selective agents. However, conjunctivitis, a known side effect, is less common in IL-13 selective agents compared to dupilumab since they do not block type-1 receptors. Progressive efficacy and off-treatment response duration of anti-OX40/OX40L are promising and different from current therapy modalities. At present, guidelines for systemic therapies do not clearly state which treatment should be used in which order. Therefore, in severe cases, where improving symptoms and quality of life are more important than the uncertain serious side effects that the agent may cause, JAKi may be preferred, whereas in cases where side effects are a concern because of risk factors or who have previously experienced side effects and have relatively less severe disease, biologics may be chosen.

## Acknowledgements

All figures used in this chapter were prepared with Biorender. Com.

## Conflict of interest

The authors declare no conflict of interest and no funding source.

## Author details

Muhammed Ali Mergen, Tubanur Cetinarslan* and Aylin Turel Ermertcan
Medical Faculty, Department of Dermatology and Venereology, Manisa Celal Bayar University, Manisa, Turkey

*Address all correspondence to: t_sarmis@windowslive.com

## References

[1] Weidinger S, Novak N. Atopic dermatitis. Lancet. 2016;**387**(10023):1109-1122

[2] Deckers IA, McLean S, Linssen S, Mommers M, van Schayck CP, Sheikh A. Investigating international time trends in the incidence and prevalence of atopic eczema; 1990

[3] Laughter MR, Maymone MBC, Mashayekhi S, Arents BWM, Karimkhani C, Langan SM, et al. The global burden of atopic dermatitis: Lessons from the global burden of disease study 1990-2017. British Journal of Dermatology. 2021;**184**(2):304-309

[4] Illi S, von Mutius E, Lau S, Nickel R, Grüber C, Niggemann B, et al. The natural course of atopic dermatitis from birth to age 7 years and the association with asthma. The Journal of Allergy and Clinical Immunology. 2004;**113**(5):925-931

[5] Garmhausen D, Hagemann T, Bieber T, Dimitriou I, Fimmers R, Diepgen T, et al. Characterization of different courses of atopic dermatitis in adolescent and adult patients. Allergy. 2013;**68**(4):498-506

[6] Fishbein AB, Silverberg JI, Wilson EJ, Ong PY. Update on atopic dermatitis: Diagnosis, severity assessment, and treatment selection. The Journal of Allergy and Clinical Immunology. In Practice. 2020;**8**(1):91-101

[7] Neri I, Galli E, Baiardini I, Picozza M, Rossi AB, Matruglio P, et al. Implications of atopic dermatitis on the quality of life of 6-11 years old children and caregivers (PEDI-BURDEN). The Journal of Asthma and Allergy. 2023;**12**(16):383-396

[8] Weidinger S, Beck LA, Bieber T, Kabashima K, Irvine AD. Atopic dermatitis. Nature Reviews Disease Primers. 2018;**4**(1):1

[9] Kapur S, Watson W, Carr S. Atopic dermatitis. Allergy asthma. Clinical Immunology. 2018;**14**(Suppl. 2):52

[10] Boguniewicz M, Leung DY. Atopic dermatitis: A disease of altered skin barrier and immune dysregulation. Immunological Reviews. 2011;**242**(1):233-246

[11] Leung DY. New insights into atopic dermatitis: Role of skin barrier and immune dysregulation. Allergology International. 2013;**62**(2):151-161

[12] Pareek A, Kumari L, Pareek A, Chaudhary S, Ratan Y, Janmeda P, et al. Unraveling atopic dermatitis: Insights into pathophysiology, therapeutic advances, and future perspectives. Cells. 2024;**13**(5):425

[13] Thapa B, Kato S, Nishizaki D, et al. OX40/OX40 ligand and its role in precision immune oncology. Cancer Metastasis Reviews. 2024;**43**:1001-1013

[14] Croft M. Co-stimulatory members of the TNFR family: Keys to effective T-cell immunity? Nature Reviews. Immunology. 2003;**3**(8):609-620

[15] Weidinger S, Bieber T, Cork MJ, Reich A, Wilson R, Quaratino S, et al. Safety and efficacy of amlitelimab, a fully human nondepleting, noncytotoxic anti-OX40 ligand monoclonal antibody, in atopic dermatitis: Results of a phase IIa randomized placebo-controlled trial. The British Journal of Dermatology. 2023;**189**(5):531-539

[16] Lé AM, Torres T. OX40-OX40L inhibition for the treatment of atopic dermatitis-focus on Rocatinlimab and Amlitelimab. Pharmaceutics. 2022;**14**(12):2753

[17] Rewerska B, Sher LD, Alpizar S, Pauser S, Pulka G, Mozaffarian N, et al. Phase 2b randomized trial of OX40 inhibitor telazorlimab for moderate-to-severe atopic dermatitis. The Journal of Allergy and Clinical Immunology. 2023;**3**(1):100195

[18] Furue M. Regulation of skin barrier function via competition between AHR Axis versus IL-13/IL-4–JAK–STAT6/STAT3 Axis: Pathogenic and therapeutic implications in atopic dermatitis. Journal of Clinical Medicine. 2020;**9**(11):3741

[19] Dubin C, Del Duca E, Guttman-Yassky E. The IL-4, IL-13 and IL-31 pathways in atopic dermatitis. Expert Review of Clinical Immunology. 2021;**17**(8):835-852

[20] Oetjen LK, Mack MR, Feng J, Whelan TM, Niu H, Guo CJ, et al. Sensory neurons Co-opt classical immune Signaling pathways to mediate chronic itch. Cell. 2017;**171**(1):217-228.e13

[21] Datsi A, Steinhoff M, Ahmad F, Alam M, Buddenkotte J. Interleukin-31: The "itchy" cytokine in inflammation and therapy. Allergy. 2021;**76**(10):2982-2997

[22] Hamilton JD, Harel S, Swanson BN, Brian W, Chen Z, Rice MS, et al. Dupilumab suppresses type 2 inflammatory biomarkers across multiple atopic, allergic diseases. Clinical and Experimental Allergy. 2021;**51**(7):915-931

[23] Wollenberg A, Weidinger S, Worm M, Bieber T. Tralokinumab in atopic dermatitis. Journal der Deutschen Dermatologischen Gesellschaft. 2021;**19**(10):1435-1442

[24] Guttman-Yassky E, Blauvelt A, Eichenfield LF, Paller AS, Armstrong AW, Drew J, et al. Efficacy and safety of Lebrikizumab, a high-affinity interleukin 13 inhibitor, in adults with moderate to severe atopic dermatitis: A phase 2b randomized clinical trial. JAMA Dermatology. 2020;**156**(4):411-420

[25] Cevikbas F, Ward A, Veverka KA. Eblasakimab, an anti-IL 13Rα1 antibody, reduces atopy-associated serum biomarkers in moderate to severe atopic dermatitis. BioDrugs. 2024;**38**(6):821-830

[26] Kwatra SG, Yosipovitch G, Legat FJ, Reich A, Paul C, Simon D, et al. Ständer S; OLYMPIA 2 investigators. Phase 3 trial of Nemolizumab in patients with Prurigo Nodularis. The New England Journal of Medicine. 2023;**389**(17):1579-1589

[27] Eichenfield LF, Tom WL, Chamlin SL, Feldman SR, Hanifin JM, Simpson EL, et al. Guidelines of care for the management of atopic dermatitis: Section 1. Diagnosis and assessment of atopic dermatitis. Journal of the American Academy of Dermatology. 2014;**70**(2):338-351

[28] Severity scoring of atopic dermatitis: The SCORAD index. Consensus report of the European task force on atopic dermatitis. Dermatology. 1993;**186**(1):23-31. DOI: 10.1159/000247298

[29] Simpson E, Bissonnette R, Eichenfield LF, Guttman-Yassky E, King B, Silverberg JI, et al. The validated investigator global assessment for atopic dermatitis (vIGA-AD): The development and reliability testing of a novel clinical outcome measurement instrument for the severity of atopic dermatitis.

Journal of the American Academy of Dermatology. 2020;**83**(3):839-846

[30] Hanifin JM, Thurston M, Omoto M, Cherill R, Tofte SJ, Graeber M. The eczema area and severity index (EASI): Assessment of reliability in atopic dermatitis. Experimental Dermatology. 2001;**10**(1):11-18

[31] Wollenberg A, Kinberger M, Arents B, Aszodi N, Avila Valle G, Barbarot S, et al. European guideline (EuroGuiDerm) on atopic eczema: Part I - systemic therapy. Journal of the European Academy of Dermatology and Venereology. 2022;**36**(9):1409-1431

[32] Davis DMR, Drucker AM, Alikhan A, Bercovitch L, Cohen DE, Darr JM, et al. Guidelines of care for the management of atopic dermatitis in adults with phototherapy and systemic therapies. Journal of the American Academy of Dermatology. 2024;**90**(2):e43-e56

[33] Lytvyn Y, Gooderham M. Targeting interleukin 13 for the treatment of atopic dermatitis. Pharmaceutics. 2023;**15**(2):568

[34] Dupixent (Dupilumab) Injection, for Subcutaneous Use. US FDA Approved Product Information. Tarrytown, NY: Regeneron Pharmaceuticals; 2022

[35] European Medicines Agency. Dupixent (dupilumab) summary of product characteristics [Accessed: August 3, 2023]

[36] Silverberg JI, Yosipovitch G, Simpson EL, Kim BS, Wu JJ, Eckert L, et al. Dupilumab treatment results in early and sustained improvements in itch in adolescents and adults with moderate to severe atopic dermatitis: Analysis of the randomized phase 3 studies SOLO 1 and SOLO 2, AD ADOL, and CHRONOS. Journal of the American Academy of Dermatology. 2020;**82**(6):1328-1336

[37] Blauvelt A, de Bruin-Weller M, Gooderham M, Cather JC, Weisman J, Pariser D, et al. Long-term management of moderate-to-severe atopic dermatitis with dupilumab and concomitant topical corticosteroids (LIBERTY AD CHRONOS): A 1-year, randomised, double-blinded, placebo-controlled, phase 3 trial. Lancet. 2017;**389**(10086):2287-2303

[38] Simpson EL, Paller AS, Siegfried EC, Boguniewicz M, Sher L, Gooderham MJ, et al. Efficacy and safety of dupilumab in adolescents with uncontrolled moderate to severe atopic dermatitis: A Phase 3 Randomized Clinical Trial. JAMA Dermatology. 2020;**156**(1):44-56

[39] Paller AS, Simpson EL, Siegfried EC, Cork MJ, Wollenberg A, Arkwright PD, et al. Dupilumab in children aged 6 months to younger than 6 years with uncontrolled atopic dermatitis: A randomised, double-blind, placebo-controlled, phase 3 trial. Lancet. 2022;**400**(10356):908-919

[40] Kreeshan FC, Al-Janabi A, Warren RB, Hunter HJA. Real-world experience and laboratory monitoring of Dupilumab in patients with moderate to severe atopic dermatitis in a tertiary Centre. Dermatology and Therapy. 2021;**11**(1):149-160

[41] Paller AS, Siegfried EC, Cork MJ, Wollenberg A, Arkwright PD, Gonzalez ME, et al. Laboratory safety from a randomized 16-week phase III study of Dupilumab in children aged 6 months to 5 years with moderate-to-severe atopic dermatitis. Paediatric Drugs. 2023;**25**(1):67-77

[42] Siegfried EC, Bieber T, Simpson EL, Paller AS, Beck LA, Boguniewicz M,

et al. Effect of Dupilumab on laboratory parameters in adolescents with atopic dermatitis: Results from a randomized, placebo-controlled, phase 3 clinical trial. American Journal of Clinical Dermatology. 2021;**22**(2):243-255

[43] Narla S, Silverberg JI, Simpson EL. Management of inadequate response and adverse effects to dupilumab in atopic dermatitis. Journal of the American Academy of Dermatology. 2022;**86**(3):628-636

[44] Fachler T, Shreberk-Hassidim R, Molho-Pessach V. Dupilumab-induced ocular surface disease: A systematic review. Journal of the American Academy of Dermatology. 2022;**86**(2): 486-487

[45] Guex-Crosier Y, Di-Lucca J, Häusermann P, Laffitte E, Saulite I, Schmid-Grendelmeier P, et al. Management of dupilumab-associated ocular surface diseases in atopic dermatitis patients. Swiss Medical Weekly. 2021;**20**(151):w30020

[46] Shi VY, Chamberlain W, Siegfried E, Kraff-Cooper C, Beckman K, Lio P, et al. Practical management of ocular surface disease in patients with atopic dermatitis, with a focus on conjunctivitis: A review. Journal of the American Academy of Dermatology. 2023;**89**(2):309-315

[47] Agnihotri G, Shi K, Lio PA. A Clinician's guide to the recognition and management of Dupilumab-associated conjunctivitis. Drugs in R&D. 2019;**19**(4):311-318

[48] Jo CE, Finstad A, Georgakopoulos JR, Piguet V, Yeung J, Drucker AM. Facial and neck erythema associated with dupilumab treatment: A systematic review. Journal of the American Academy of Dermatology. 2021;**84**(5):1339-1347

[49] Jay R, Rodger J, Zirwas M. Review of dupilumab-associated inflammatory arthritis: An approach to clinical analysis and management. JAAD Case Reports. 2022;**6**(21):14-18

[50] Lobo Y, Lee RC, Spelman L. Atopic dermatitis treated safely with Dupilumab during pregnancy: A case report and review of the literature. Case Reports in Dermatology. 2021;**13**(2):248-256

[51] Deleuran M, Dézfoulian B, Elberling J, Knutar I, Lapeere H, Lossius AH, et al. Systemic anti-inflammatory treatment of atopic dermatitis during conception, pregnancy and breastfeeding: Interdisciplinary expert consensus in northern Europe. Journal of the European Academy of Dermatology and Venereology. 2024;**38**(1):31-41

[52] Lockhart MK, Siegfried EC. Evolving landscape of systemic therapy for Pediatric atopic dermatitis. Dermatologic Clinics. 2022;**40**(2):137-143

[53] Blauvelt A, Teixeira HD, Simpson EL, Costanzo A, De Bruin-Weller M, Barbarot S, et al. Efficacy and safety of Upadacitinib vs Dupilumab in adults with moderate-to-severe atopic dermatitis: A randomized clinical trial. JAMA Dermatology. 2021;**157**(9):1047-1055

[54] Bieber T, Simpson EL, Silverberg JI, Thaçi D, Paul C, Pink AE, et al. Abrocitinib versus placebo or Dupilumab for atopic dermatitis. The New England Journal of Medicine. 2021;**384**(12):1101-1112

[55] Drucker AM, Morra DE, Prieto-Merino D, Ellis AG, Yiu ZZN, Rochwerg B, et al. Systemic immunomodulatory treatments for atopic dermatitis: Update of a living systematic review and network

meta-analysis. JAMA Dermatology. 2022;**158**(5):523-532

[56] Adbry® (tralokinumab-ldrm) Prescribing Information. LEO Pharma; 2024

[57] European Medicines Agency. Tralokinumab: EU summary of product characteristics and assessment report; 2021

[58] Wollenberg A, Blauvelt A, Guttman-Yassky E, Worm M, Lynde C, Lacour JP, et al. ECZTRA 1 and ECZTRA 2 study investigators. Tralokinumab for moderate-to-severe atopic dermatitis: Results from two 52-week, randomized, double-blind, multicentre, placebo-controlled phase III trials (ECZTRA 1 and ECZTRA 2). The British Journal of Dermatology. 2021;**184**(3):437-449

[59] Silverberg JI, Toth D, Bieber T, Alexis AF, Elewski BE, Pink AE, et al. ECZTRA 3 study investigators. Tralokinumab plus topical corticosteroids for the treatment of moderate-to-severe atopic dermatitis: Results from the double-blind, randomized, multicentre, placebo-controlled phase III ECZTRA 3 trial. The British Journal of Dermatology. 2021;**184**(3):450-463

[60] Paller AS, Flohr C, Cork M, Bewley A, Blauvelt A, Hong HC, et al. Efficacy and safety of Tralokinumab in adolescents with moderate to severe atopic dermatitis: The phase 3 ECZTRA 6 randomized clinical trial. JAMA Dermatology. 2023;**159**(6):596-605

[61] Simpson EL, Merola JF, Silverberg JI, Reich K, Warren RB, Staumont-Sallé D, et al. Safety of tralokinumab in adult patients with moderate-to-severe atopic dermatitis: Pooled analysis of five randomized, double-blind, placebo-controlled phase II and phase III trials. The British Journal of Dermatology. 2022;**187**(6):888-899

[62] Paller A, Cork M, Hong C-h, Soong W, Schneider S, Lo H, et al. 549- laboratory parameters in adolescent patients aged 12-17 with moderate-to-severe atopic dermatitis treated with tralokinumab up to week 52: Results from the phase 3 ECZTRA 6 trial. British Journal of Dermatology. 2024;**190**(Suppl. 2):ii47-ii48

[63] Doran E, Cai F, Holweg CTJ, Wong K, Brumm J, Arron JR. Interleukin-13 in asthma and other eosinophilic disorders. Frontiers in Medicine. 2017;**4**:139

[64] Shakuntulla F, Chiarella SE. Safety of biologics for atopic diseases during pregnancy. The Journal of Allergy and Clinical Immunology. In Practice. 2022;**10**(12):3149-3155

[65] EBGLYSS. Prescribing Information. Lilly USA, LLC

[66] European Medicines Agency. Lebrikizumab: EU summary of product characteristics and assessment report; 2023. Available at: https://www.ema.europa.eu/ [Accessed: December 6, 2023]

[67] Silverberg JI, Guttman-Yassky E, Thaçi D, Irvine AD, Stein Gold L, Blauvelt A, et al. ADvocate1 and ADvocate2 investigators. Two phase 3 trials of Lebrikizumab for moderate-to-severe atopic dermatitis. The New England Journal of Medicine. 2023;**388**(12):1080-1091

[68] Simpson EL, Gooderham M, Wollenberg A, Weidinger S, Armstrong A, Soung J, et al. ADhere investigators. Efficacy and safety of Lebrikizumab in combination with topical corticosteroids in adolescents and adults with moderate-to-severe

atopic dermatitis: A randomized clinical trial (ADhere). JAMA Dermatology. 2023;**159**(2):182-191

[69] Blauvelt A, Thyssen JP, Guttman-Yassky E, Bieber T, Serra-Baldrich E, Simpson E, et al. Efficacy and safety of lebrikizumab in moderate-to-severe atopic dermatitis: 52-week results of two randomized double-blinded placebo-controlled phase III trials. The British Journal of Dermatology. 2023;**188**(6):740-748

[70] Cevikbas F, Wang X, Akiyama T, Kempkes C, Savinko T, Antal A, et al. A sensory neuron-expressed IL-31 receptor mediates T helper cell-dependent itch: Involvement of TRPV1 and TRPA1. The Journal of Allergy and Clinical Immunology. 2014;**133**(2):448-460

[71] Silverberg JI, Pinter A, Pulka G, Poulin Y, Bouaziz JD, Wollenberg A, et al. Phase 2B randomized study of nemolizumab in adults with moderate-to-severe atopic dermatitis and severe pruritus. The Journal of Allergy and Clinical Immunology. 2020;**145**(1):173-182

[72] Nemluvio. Prescribing information for atopic dermatitis. U.S. Approval; 2024

[73] Silverberg JI, Wollenberg A, Reich A, Thaçi D, Legat FJ, Papp KA, et al. ARCADIA 1 and ARCADIA 2 study investigators. Nemolizumab with concomitant topical therapy in adolescents and adults with moderate-to-severe atopic dermatitis (ARCADIA 1 and ARCADIA 2): Results from two replicate, double-blind, randomised controlled phase 3 trials. Lancet. 2024;**404**(10451):445-460

[74] Kabashima K, Matsumura T, Komazaki H, Kawashima M, Nemolizumab-JP01 Study Group. Trial of Nemolizumab and topical agents for atopic dermatitis with pruritus. The New England Journal of Medicine. 2020;**383**(2):141-150

[75] Kabashima K, Matsumura T, Komazaki H, Kawashima M, Nemolizumab JP01 and JP02 Study Group. Nemolizumab plus topical agents in patients with atopic dermatitis (AD) and moderate-to-severe pruritus provide improvement in pruritus and signs of AD for up to 68 weeks: Results from two phase III, long-term studies. The British Journal of Dermatology. 2022;**186**(4):642-651

[76] Veverka KA, Thng STG, Silverberg JI, Armstrong AW, Menezes J, Kaoukhov A, et al. Safety and efficacy of eblasakimab, an interleukin 13 receptor α1 monoclonal antibody, in adults with moderate-to-severe atopic dermatitis: A phase 1b, multiple-ascending dose study. Journal of the American Academy of Dermatology. 2024;**90**(3):504-511

[77] Simpson E, Gooderham M, Kircik L, Armstrong A, Schlesinger T, Del Rosso JQ, et al. 53652 efficacy and safety of eblasakimab in adults with severe atopic dermatitis: A posthoc analysis of the phase 2b TREK-AD trial. Journal of the American Academy of Dermatology. 2024;**91**(3) Supplement, AB194-AB194

[78] Worm M, Simpson EL, Thaçi D, et al. Efficacy and safety of multiple dupilumab dose regimens after initial successful treatment in patients with atopic dermatitis: A randomized clinical trial. JAMA Dermatology. 2020;**156**:131-143

[79] Guttman-Yassky E, Simpson EL, Reich K, Kabashima K, Igawa K, Suzuki T, et al. An anti-OX40 antibody to treat moderate-to-severe atopic dermatitis: A multicentre, double-blind, placebo-controlled phase 2b study. Lancet. 2023;**401**(10372):204-214

[80] Silverberg JI, de Bruin-Weller M, Bieber T, et al. Upadacitinib plus topical corticosteroids in atopic dermatitis: Week 52 AD up study results. The Journal of Allergy and Clinical Immunology. 2022;**149**:977-987.e14

[81] Blauvelt A, Silverberg JI, Lynde CW, et al. Abrocitinib induction, randomized withdrawal, and retreatment in patients with moderateto-severe atopic dermatitis: Results from the JAK1 atopic dermatitis efficacy and safety (JADE) REGIMEN phase 3 trial. Journal of the American Academy of Dermatology. 2022;**86**:104-112

[82] Guttman-Yassky E, Pavel AB, Zhou L, Estrada YD, Zhang N, Xu H, et al. GBR 830, an anti-OX40, improves skin gene signatures and clinical scores in patients with atopic dermatitis. The Journal of Allergy and Clinical Immunology. 2019;**144**(2):482-493.e7

Chapter 3

# Phototherapy in Atopic Dermatitis Management

*Amr Molla*


## Abstract

This chapter provides a comprehensive overview of phototherapy as a critical therapeutic option in managing atopic dermatitis (AD). AD is a chronic inflammatory skin condition characterized by a disrupted skin barrier and immune dysregulation, affecting patients' quality of life significantly. Phototherapy, particularly narrowband UVB (NB-UVB) and UVA1, has emerged as an effective approach for cases resistant to conventional treatments, offering substantial benefits in terms of safety and efficacy. This chapter examines the mechanisms by which phototherapy modulates immune responses and repairs the skin barrier, reducing inflammation and alleviating symptoms in AD. Various phototherapy modalities, including NB-UVB, broadband UVB (BB-UVB), UVA/UVB combinations, and PUVA, are explored in terms of their therapeutic advantages, optimal dosing strategies, and potential side effects. Emphasis is placed on practical considerations for clinical application, along with current research insights and areas for future study. The chapter aims to enhance clinicians' understanding of phototherapy's role in AD treatment, advocating for its broader adoption and precise application to improve patient outcomes.


**Keywords:** atopic dermatitis, phototherapy, narrowband UVB, broadband UVB, UVA, PUVA

## 1. Introduction

Atopic dermatitis (AD) is a chronic inflammatory skin disorder that significantly affects patients' quality of life. Its prevalence differs based on geographic and socioeconomic factors [1, 2]. AD appears to have a multifactorial etiology, involving genetic, environmental, and immunological factors. The etiology of AD is multifactorial, influenced by genetic, environmental, and immunological factors. In developed nations, AD is reported in 10–20% of children and 1–3% of adults, whereas in developing countries, it is less common, affecting 1–10% of children and less than 1% of adults. These differences underscore the impact of regional and environmental factors on the prevalence of the disease. Recognizing these distinctions is crucial for formulating tailored management strategies suited to specific regions for AD [3].

The primary aim of treating AD is to achieve effective disease control by reducing skin inflammation, managing pruritus, and improving patients' quality of life through personalized, long-term therapeutic strategies [1]. Treatment approaches need to consider factors such as patient age, behavior, socioeconomic background, adherence to treatments, and psychological well-being [4]. Many patients benefit from initial treatments, including gentle skin care, emollients, and allergen avoidance. However, systemic therapies may be required for those with more severe cases. Phototherapy is particularly valuable in managing acute flare-ups and chronic cases of AD that do not respond adequately to topical treatments [5].

Phototherapy is widely recognized as a second-line treatment when conventional and topical options are ineffective and applicable to both chronic and acute AD in children and adults [3]. In cases of severe, widespread AD, phototherapy may even serve as a first-line intervention. This approach uses non-ionizing radiation, specifically within the ultraviolet (UV) spectrum, to relieve symptoms [6]. Despite advancements in biological therapies, UV phototherapy remains a reliable, cost-effective, and effective treatment for inflammatory skin conditions like AD, which are marked by T-cell-rich infiltrates [1, 2].

The objective of this chapter is to provide dermatologists and clinicians with a comprehensive overview of phototherapy as a core therapeutic option in the treatment of AD, along with considerations for its integration within the broader AD management framework. Given the absence of large-scale randomized controlled studies and a definitive conclusion on the superiority of any single phototherapy modality [7], it is essential to highlight the established efficacy and safety of phototherapy. Emphasizing these aspects aims to inform clinical practice and enhance patient and clinician understanding of phototherapy's role in AD management.

## 2. Underlying mechanisms of phototherapy

The fundamental treatment approach for AD involves non-pharmacological measures, including trigger avoidance and the use of emollients to maintain skin hydration and barrier function. Topical medications such as glucocorticoids and immunomodulators prove effective for mild cases, whereas severe or treatment-resistant cases may necessitate systemic approaches like short-term use of glucocorticoids or cyclosporine in conjunction with topical treatments and hydration. Phototherapy serves as a secondary option for AD treatment. Despite limited reporting of short- and long-term adverse events, phototherapy remains a valuable therapeutic choice with a favorable efficacy and safety profile.

Phototherapy is a medical treatment utilizing specific light wavelengths to address skin conditions, either independently or in conjunction with other medications. Two primary types of phototherapy exist: ultraviolet (UV) therapy and visible light therapy. UV therapy employs UV wavelengths to treat skin disorders such as psoriasis and AD, while visible light therapy targets specific visible light wavelengths for conditions like acne and seasonal affective disorder (SAD) [8–10].

UV phototherapy acts locally, avoiding the adverse effects of profound systemic immunosuppression. It remains an essential tool for dermatologists despite the availability of biological agents. UV radiation effects can be categorized into immediate and delayed effects. Immediate effects involve damage to cellular membranes and DNA, activation of cytoplasmic transcription factors, and the isomerization of chromophores like urocanic acid, leading to immediate growth arrest and programmed cell death known as apoptosis [11, 12].

Ultraviolet radiation utilized in phototherapy interacts with cellular structures, causing targeted damage that disrupts pathogenic immune responses. UV radiation can alter DNA structures directly, leading to growth arrest and apoptosis, particularly in T cells and keratinocytes, known as phototype I reaction. These changes reduce inflammation and immune system hyperactivity, which are central to the pathology of AD [8, 10, 12].

The delayed impact of UV radiation involves suppressing the immune system by impairing the function of both adaptive and innate immune cells. This leads to the death of T cells in the skin and a reduction in the number of Langerhans cells. UV radiation also triggers T regulatory cells, which mitigate excessive immune responses. Additionally, photo-oxidative stress caused by UV radiation damages the cytoskeleton in remaining dendritic cells, inhibiting T-cell stimulation. This immune system suppression is accompanied by decreased production of inflammatory cytokines such as IL-2, IL-9, IL-17, IL-22, IL-23, IL-5, IL-13, IL-31, TNF-alpha, and TNF-gamma, while stimulating the production of IL-10, known for its immunosuppressive effect. Regarding apoptosis, UV light triggers two distinct processes. UVA1 irradiation induces immediate pre-programmed cell death and early membrane rupture through structural and functional modifications, while UVB irradiation causes DNA damage followed by delayed apoptosis with initial membrane alteration [8, 10, 12].

In addition to its impact on the immune system, ultraviolet (UV) rays can influence the function of the outermost layer of the skin, known as the epidermal barrier. UV rays have several effects on the skin:

1. Thickening of the stratum corneum: UV rays can lead to the thickening of the stratum corneum, the outermost layer of the epidermis. This thickening makes the skin less vulnerable to irritants and reduces the risk of eczematous flare-ups [8].

2. Increased expression of barrier proteins: UV rays can increase the expression of barrier proteins like filaggrin and involucrum, which are essential for maintaining the skin's integrity and protective function. These proteins contribute to the skin's ability to act as a barrier against environmental factors and help prevent moisture loss [3, 11].

3. Antibacterial properties: Studies have shown that both UVB and UVA rays have antibacterial properties, particularly against *Staphylococcus aureus*, a bacterium commonly associated with skin infections. UV radiation can decrease the bacterial count on the skin and suppress the production of toxins by bacteria, contributing to improved skin health [13].

4. UV radiation also has an impact on the production of vitamin D, a fat-soluble vitamin synthesized in the skin when UVB rays convert 7-dehydrocholesterol into pre-vitamin D. This process occurs in the uppermost skin layer. Vitamin D is then transported through the bloodstream and undergoes metabolic processes in the liver and kidneys to become its active form, 1,25-dihydroxy vitamin D (calcitriol). It has been observed that patients with atopic dermatitis (AD) often have insufficient levels of vitamin D, which can play a role in the inflammatory process and potentially lead to defects in the epidermal barrier [14].

When determining the appropriate dose and treatment schedule for phototherapy, various factors need to be considered, including the severity of the condition, the patient's overall health, the cost of treatment, accessibility to care, the location and phototype (skin type) of the affected skin lesions, any history of skin cancer, photosensitivity history, the Fitzpatrick skin type (a classification system for human skin color), and the least erythema dose (a measure of the skin's response to UV exposure) [5]. For patients with refractory or chronic diseases, phototherapy can be administered on a regular but intermittent basis over time, or it may be used more continuously as maintenance therapy [15].

Despite its effectiveness in treating AD, phototherapy does have limitations. One of these limitations is the requirement for bi-weekly sessions, which can be challenging for patients who live far from medical centers with phototherapy technology. Additionally, not all individuals may benefit from phototherapy, and those with light-sensitive conditions may not be suitable candidates for this treatment. Furthermore, different types of phototherapy carry varying levels of risk, which clinicians must carefully consider when selecting the most appropriate treatment approach [16]. Common adverse effects of phototherapy include actinic damage, local erythema, and tenderness, pruritus, burning, and stinging. Less common consequences may include non-melanoma skin cancer, melanoma (especially with PUVA therapy), lentigines, photosensitive eruptions (such as polymorphous light eruption), folliculitis, photo onycholysis, herpes simplex virus reactivation, and facial hypertrichosis. UVA therapy may lead to cataract formation, while the addition of oral psoralen to UVA treatment may cause patients to experience headaches, nausea, vomiting, and, rarely, hepatotoxicity [1, 16]. Oral psoralen can also increase a patient's photosensitivity, both cutaneous and ocular, for several hours following ingestion [16].

## 3. Clinical indications for phototherapy in atopic dermatitis

Phototherapy, a well-established therapeutic modality, has emerged as a significant treatment option for patients suffering from atopic dermatitis, particularly when conventional first-line treatments such as emollients, topical steroids, and topical calcineurin inhibitors are ineffective. Atopic dermatitis, characterized by chronic inflammation and a disrupted skin barrier, often responds favorably to phototherapy due to its multifaceted therapeutic effects. Ultraviolet (UV) light, primarily in the form of narrowband UVB (NB-UVB), is the most commonly used spectrum in phototherapy for this condition. It works by inducing immunomodulatory effects that help in reducing inflammation and pruritus associated with atopic dermatitis. Additionally, UV light helps in restoring the integrity of the skin barrier, which is compromised in atopic dermatitis patients. This restoration is achieved through the upregulation of proteins and lipids that are essential for barrier function. Moreover, phototherapy has been shown to have an antipruritic effect, which significantly improves the quality of life for patients by reducing the itch-scratch cycle, a critical factor in the exacerbation of atopic dermatitis. The treatment's effectiveness is influenced by several patient-specific factors, such as skin type, severity and extent of the disease, and the patient's previous response to other treatments. It is essential that phototherapy be administered under the guidance of a knowledgeable physician to optimize treatment parameters like the dose and schedule, tailored to the individual's needs and characteristics, and to monitor for potential side effects [1, 3, 8, 17, 18].

Therefore, phototherapy is a recognized treatment option for AD when standard therapies fail. The following recommendations guide its application:

1. Employ phototherapy when first-line treatments, including emollients, topical corticosteroids, and calcineurin inhibitors, prove insufficient.

2. Consider phototherapy as a long-term management option for chronic, persistent AD cases.

3. Ensure phototherapy is administered under the supervision of a clinician who is experienced in its use.

4. Factors in patient-specific considerations, include accessibility, cost, skin type, history of photosensitivity, and any previous skin cancer.

5. Tailor the phototherapy schedule to the patient's minimal erythema dose (MED) or Fitzpatrick skin type for safe and effective treatment.

6. Evaluate home phototherapy as an alternative for patients unable to access clinic-based care, with appropriate monitoring by a healthcare provider.

## 4. Therapeutic phototherapy methods in atopic dermatitis

Phototherapy, or photochemotherapy, when combined with psoralens, represents a valuable treatment option for AD. Various phototherapy types utilize specific light wavelengths to address AD and other skin conditions, helping to alleviate symptoms and reduce disease activity. Below are some key phototherapy modalities used in treating AD.

### 4.1 Narrowband UVB and broadband UVB

Narrowband UVB (NB-UVB) and broadband UVB (BB-UVB) are two primary forms of ultraviolet B light therapy used in dermatology, particularly for treating inflammatory skin conditions like atopic dermatitis. NB-UVB emits a specific, narrow wavelength range of 311–313 nm, which has been shown to be effective in reducing skin inflammation while minimizing adverse effects compared to broader UV ranges. This targeted wavelength enables NB-UVB to suppress immune pathways involved in atopic dermatitis, including Th2, Th22, and Th1 responses, making it the preferred choice due to its favorable safety and efficacy profile [17, 19]. Dosing guidelines for narrowband ultraviolet B are shown in **Table 1**.

The therapeutic application of phototherapy in atopic dermatitis depends on determining optimal dosing strategies, particularly through minimal erythema doses (MEDs). MEDs, the minimum light exposure required to cause visible reddening of the skin, serve as the initial benchmark for treatment dosage. Doses are adjusted to each patient, with adjustments based on skin type and individual response to maximize efficacy and minimize adverse effects [20]. The variability in MEDs for narrowband UVB (NB-UVB) across different skin types necessitates routine MED testing and regular calibration of the UVB machine, ideally on a weekly basis, to account for the gradual decline in lamp efficacy over time. Without consistent measurement and adjustment of UV output, clinicians may unintentionally deliver lower-than-intended doses, which could impact treatment outcomes. Safety measures, including dose adjustments, patient education, and routine skin assessments, are critical to reduce risks and enhance patient satisfaction. The frequency of phototherapy sessions required for effective maintenance differs for each patient; while a gradual decrease in frequency is ideal, some individuals may require ongoing weekly NB-UVB sessions

| Skin types | Initial UVB dose ($mJ/cm^2$) | UVB increase after each treatment ($mJ/cm^2$) | Maximum dose ($mJ/cm^2$) |
|---|---|---|---|
| *According to skin type:* | | | |
| I | 130 | 15 | 2000 |
| II | 220 | 25 | 2000 |
| III | 260 | 40 | 3000 |
| IV | 330 | 45 | 3000 |
| V | 350 | 60 | 5000 |
| VI | 400 | 65 | 5000 |
| *According to MED:* | | | |
| Initial UVB | | 50% of MED | |
| Treatments 1–20 | | Increase by 10% of initial MED | |
| Treatment ≥21 | | Increase as ordered by physician | |
| *If subsequent treatments are missed for:* | | | |
| 4–7 days | | Keep dose same | |
| 1–2 weeks | | Decrease dose by 25% | |
| 2–3 weeks | | Decrease dose by 50% or start over | |
| 3–4 weeks | | Start over | |
| *Maintenance therapy for NB-UVB after > 95% clearance:* | | | |
| 1×/week | NB-UVB for 4 weeks | Keep dose same | |
| 1×/2 weeks | NB-UVB for 4 weeks | Decrease dose by 25% | |
| 1×/4 weeks | NB-UVB | 50% of highest dose | |

**Table 1.**
*Dosing guidelines for narrowband ultraviolet B (administered 3–5×/week).*

to sustain long-term effectiveness. Accurate MED dosing and careful maintenance are essential for achieving optimal treatment outcomes in clinical settings [7].

In contrast, BB-UVB emits a broader range of wavelengths (290–320 nm), which includes more of the shorter UVB rays that can increase the risk of erythema (skin redness) and other side effects. While BB-UVB can still be effective, it is generally considered less optimal than NB-UVB, particularly for sensitive or extensive AD cases [1, 3, 7, 8, 18]. Dosing guidelines for broadband ultraviolet B are presented in **Table 2** [17, 19].

## 4.2 Combined UVA/UVB

Combined UVA/UVB therapy uses a single device to emit both UVA and UVB radiation, covering a wavelength range from 280 to 400 nm. This modality allows for simultaneous or sequential exposure to both types of UV light, capitalizing on the benefits of each. UVB, known for its ability to reduce inflammation by penetrating the outer layers of the skin, works effectively on active lesions and acute flares. Meanwhile, UVA penetrates deeper into the skin, targeting the dermal layers to suppress the immune cells involved in chronic inflammation. Combined UVA/UVB therapy is particularly useful in patients with widespread or severe atopic dermatitis,

| Skin types | Initial UVB dose (mJ/cm$^2$) | UVB increase after each treatment (mJ/cm$^2$) |
|---|---|---|
| *According to skin type:* | | |
| I | 20 | 5 |
| II | 25 | 10 |
| III | 30 | 15 |
| IV | 40 | 20 |
| V | 50 | 25 |
| VI | 60 | 30 |
| *According to MED:* | | |
| Initial UVB | 50% of MED | |
| Treatments 1–10 | Increase by 25% of initial MED | |
| Treatments 11–20 | Increase by 10% of initial MED | |
| Treatment ≥21 | Increase as ordered by physician | |
| *If subsequent treatments are missed for:* | | |
| 4–7 days | Keep dose same | |
| 1–2 weeks | Decrease dose by 50% | |
| 2–3 weeks | Decrease dose by 75% | |
| 3–4 weeks | Start over | |

**Table 2.**
*Dosing guidelines for broadband ultraviolet B (administered 3–5×/week).*

though it is used less frequently today due to the limited availability of combination devices and the more refined efficacy of specific phototherapy types, such as narrowband UVB [1, 3, 6–8, 18, 19].

### 4.3 UVA and UVA-1

UVA therapy, especially UVA-1 (340–400 nm), focuses solely on long-wavelength ultraviolet A light, which can penetrate deeper into the skin compared to UVB. UVA-1 is particularly beneficial for treating chronic inflammatory skin conditions like atopic dermatitis, as it modulates deeper immune responses and reduces skin inflammation by affecting T-cell activity and cytokine production. UVA-1 is typically administered in varying doses—high, medium, or low—depending on the severity and extent of the skin condition. Compared to traditional UVA, which spans a broader range, UVA-1 targets a narrower spectrum that maximizes therapeutic effects while minimizing potential adverse effects, making it a versatile option in managing persistent or chronic cases of AD [1, 3, 6–8, 18, 19].

### 4.4 PUVA (psoralens and UVA)

PUVA therapy is often a secondary choice for AD treatment. It involves combining psoralens (8-methoxy psoralen) with synthetic long-wave ultraviolet A (UVA) radiation. Psoralens can be administered orally (systemic PUVA), topically (cream-PUVA), or via water (balneotherapy) [19].

| Skin types | Initial dose (J/cm²) | Increments (J/cm²) | Maximum dose (J/cm²) |
|---|---|---|---|
| I | 0.5 | 0.5 | 8 |
| II | 1.0 | 0.5 | 8 |
| III | 1.5 | 1.0 | 12 |
| IV | 2.0 | 1.0 | 12 |
| V | 2.5 | 1.5 | 20 |
| VI | 3.0 | 1.5 | 20 |

**Table 3.**
*Dosing of UVA radiation for oral psoralen plus ultraviolet A.*

The mechanism of PUVA involves inducing DNA damage, depleting nucleotides in peripheral blood leukocytes, and triggering polyADP-ribosylation, leading to T-cell death. Recent studies indicate that PUVA treatment may reduce itching and clinical severity in AD patients by regulating epidermal nerve density and modifying the expression of specific axonal molecules such as semaphorin 3A (Sema3A) and nerve growth factor (NGF). However, PUVA should be used cautiously due to its potential carcinogenic effects with long-term use [1, 3, 6, 8, 18]. Dosing for oral psoralen plus UVA is provided in **Table 3** [17, 19].

## 5. Conclusion

In conclusion, this chapter has illuminated the multifaceted nature of atopic dermatitis (AD) and the central role of phototherapy in its management. Through a thorough analysis, we have established that phototherapy, particularly modalities such as narrowband UVB (NB-UVB) and UVA1, stands out as an effective treatment option for AD, offering considerable benefits in terms of safety and efficacy. These insights emphasize the value of phototherapy within the treatment landscape for AD, especially in cases unresponsive to standard treatments.

The implications for clinical practice are substantial, supporting the broader integration of phototherapy into AD management and advocating for its earlier consideration in treatment plans to enhance patient outcomes. Additionally, our findings underscore the importance of clinicians' familiarity with various phototherapy modalities, enabling them to customize treatments to meet the specific needs of individual patients effectively.

Despite the demonstrated strengths of phototherapy, this chapter also recognizes the need for further research. Future studies should focus on:

1. Exploring the long-term safety and efficacy of phototherapy across diverse patient populations, including pediatric cases and severe AD.

2. Investigating the mechanisms that underpin the therapeutic effects of different phototherapy modalities, which could enhance our understanding and pave the way for more targeted therapies.

3. Evaluating the cost-effectiveness of phototherapy in AD management by assessing both direct treatment costs and the broader impact on patients' quality of life.

*DOI: http://dx.doi.org/10.5772/intechopen.1008797*

Addressing these research areas will allow for the refinement of phototherapy protocols, improvement of patient care, and the discovery of novel therapeutic targets within AD pathophysiology. This chapter calls for continued research to unlock the full potential of phototherapy in dermatology, ensuring that AD patients receive the most effective and individualized care possible.

## Acknowledgements

I would like to express my sincere gratitude to all the authors and researchers whose work contributed to the foundation of this chapter. Special thanks go to Dr. Muayad Albadrani for his invaluable guidance and support throughout this project. I am also grateful to the College of Medicine, Taibah University, Madinah, for providing the necessary resources and a supportive environment for completing this work. Additionally, I thank my peers and colleagues for their constructive feedback and insightful suggestions, which significantly enhanced the quality of this chapter. This contribution to the book would not have been possible without the collaborative support of the individuals and institutions mentioned above.

## Author contributions

The author, Amr Molla, took primary responsibility for conceptualizing and writing this chapter. Key contributions included conducting a thorough literature review, synthesizing research findings on phototherapy in atopic dermatitis, and analyzing its clinical applications and therapeutic advancements. The author ensured that the chapter integrates practical insights for clinicians and researchers, thoroughly revised the text for clarity and coherence, and addressed editorial feedback to enhance the overall quality.

## Funding sources

This chapter was developed without external funding. The author received no financial support or grants for this work.

## Conflict of interest

The author declares no financial or non-financial conflicts of interest that could influence the research or objectivity of this chapter.

## Acronyms and abbreviations

| | |
|---|---|
| AD | atopic dermatitis |
| UV | ultraviolet |
| ISAAC | International Study of Asthma and Allergies in Childhood |
| GDP | gross domestic product |
| Ig | immunoglobulin |

| | |
|---|---|
| FLG | filaggrin |
| LOR | loricrin |
| IVL | involucrin |
| IL | interleukin |
| TSLP | thymic stromal lymphopoietin |
| SAD | seasonal affective disorder |
| Th | T helper |
| IFN | interferon |
| NK | natural killer |
| NB-UVB | narrowband UVB |
| BB-UVB | broadband UVB |
| PUVA | psoralens and UVA |
| SCORAD | scoring atopic dermatitis |
| HD | high dose |
| MD | medium dose |
| LD | low dose |
| NGF | nerve growth factor |
| Sema3A | semaphorin 3A |
| TCS | topical corticosteroids |
| TCI | topical calcineurin inhibitors |
| PDE4 | phosphodiesterase 4 |
| NSAIDs | nonsteroidal anti-inflammatory drugs |
| MTX | methotrexate |
| JAK | Janus kinase |

## Author details

Amr Molla
Department of Medicine, College of Medicine, Taibah University, Madinah, Saudi Arabia

*Address all correspondence to: amolla@taibahu.edu.sa

## References

[1] Bolognia J et al. Dermatology. 2nd ed. Philadelphia, PA, USA: Mosby Elsevier; 2008

[2] James WD, Elston D, Berger T. Andrew's Diseases of the Skin E-Book: Clinical Dermatology. Philadelphia, PA, USA: Elsevier Health Sciences; 2011

[3] Wolff K et al. Fitzpatrick's Dermatology in General Medicine. New York: McGraw-Hill; 2008

[4] Kim JE et al. Consensus guidelines for the treatment of atopic dermatitis in Korea (part I): General management and topical treatment. Annals of Dermatology. 2015;**27**(5):563-577

[5] Davis DM et al. Atopic dermatitis: Phototherapy and systemic therapy. Seminars in Cutaneous Medicine and Surgery. 2017;**36**(3):118-123

[6] Vangipuram R, Feldman S. Ultraviolet phototherapy for cutaneous diseases: A concise review. Oral Diseases. 2016;**22**(4):253-259

[7] Patrizi A, Raone B, Ravaioli GM. Management of atopic dermatitis: Safety and efficacy of phototherapy. Clinical, Cosmetic and Investigational Dermatology. 2015;**8**:511-520

[8] Ganzetti G, Campanati A, Offidani A. Phototherapy in Dermatology. Dermatology—Laboratory and Clinical Research. Hauppauge, NY, USA: Nova Science Publishers; 2017

[9] Gambichler T. Management of atopic dermatitis using photo (chemo) therapy. Archives of Dermatological Research. 2009;**301**(3):197-203

[10] Vieyra-Garcia PA, Wolf P. A deep dive into UV-based phototherapy: Mechanisms of action and emerging molecular targets in inflammation and cancer. Pharmacology & Therapeutics. 2021;**222**:107784

[11] Borgia F et al. Oxidative stress and phototherapy in atopic dermatitis: Mechanisms, role, and future perspectives. Biomolecules. 2022;**12**(12):1904

[12] Kemény L, Varga E, Novak Z. Advances in phototherapy for psoriasis and atopic dermatitis. Expert Review of Clinical Immunology. 2019;**15**(11):1205-1214

[13] Burns EM et al. Ultraviolet radiation, both UVA and UVB, influences the composition of the skin microbiome. Experimental Dermatology. 2019;**28**(2):136-141

[14] Juzeniene A et al. Phototherapy and vitamin D. Clinics in Dermatology. 2016;**34**(5):548-555

[15] Eichenfield LF et al. Guidelines of care for the management of atopic dermatitis: Section 2. Management and treatment of atopic dermatitis with topical therapies. Journal of the American Academy of Dermatology. 2014;**71**(1):116-132

[16] Valejo Coelho MM, Apetato M. The dark side of the light: Phototherapy adverse effects. Clinics in Dermatology. 2016;**34**(5):556-562

[17] Sidbury R et al. Guidelines of care for the management of atopic dermatitis: Section 3. Management and treatment with phototherapy and systemic agents. Journal of the American Academy of Dermatology. 2014;**71**(2):327-349

[18] Dogra S, Mahajan R. Phototherapy for atopic dermatitis. Indian Journal of Dermatology, Venereology and Leprology. 2015;**81**:10

[19] Molla A. A comprehensive review of phototherapy in atopic dermatitis: Mechanisms, modalities, and clinical efficacy. Cureus. 2024;**16**(3):e56890

[20] Heckman CJ et al. Minimal erythema dose (MED) testing. Journal of Visualized Experiments. 2013;**75**:e50175

Chapter 4

# JAK Inhibitors in the Management of Atopic Dermatitis: Mechanisms, Efficacy, and Future Directions

*Mohammed Alraddadi, Abdullah Ahmed Alhejaily and Amr Molla*

## Abstract

In this chapter, we aim to provide a detailed overview of the role of Janus Kinase (JAK) inhibitors in the management of atopic dermatitis (AD). Atopic dermatitis (AD) is a chronic inflammatory skin disorder with a huge economic and health burden. The chapter will investigate the immunopathogenesis of AD with the focus on the JAK-STAT signaling pathway. Additionally, we target to demonstrate its dysregulation and its contribution to disease progression. The chapter will importantly examine the current evidence on the efficacy and safety of both selective and non-selective JAK inhibitors based on current clinical trials. Moreover, it will discuss the practical recommendations for clinical use, monitoring approaches, and patient selection principles. Emerging data, challenges, and future research directions of the long-term safety and efficacy of JAK inhibitors in the AD treatment algorithm will also be addressed. This chapter will serve as a comprehensive resource for clinicians and researchers for the targeted therapy in atopic dermatitis.

**Keywords:** atopic dermatitis, JAK inhibitors, JAK-STAT pathway, targeted therapy, immunomodulation, clinical trials, safety profile, emerging treatments

## 1. Introduction

Atopic dermatitis (AD) is a common, chronic skin disorder. It is a relapsing inflammatory condition with a substantial physical and psychological burden on patients globally. The most common symptoms of this disorder include eczematous lesions, pruritus, and skin barrier dysfunction. The pathogenesis of AD is complex interactions among genetic predisposition, environmental factors, and immune dysregulation. While traditional treatment strategies, such as topical corticosteroids, calcineurin inhibitors, and systemic immunosuppressants, provide symptomatic relief, they usually fail to achieve sustained disease control. Furthermore, most of them carry significant side effects [1]. Recently, the general understanding of AD pathophysiology has been improved. Subsequently, targeted immune pathways therapies have emerged as better potential therapies. Among these, Janus kinase (JAK) inhibitors have developed as a promising class of oral and topical agents with


IntechOpen

a possibility to modulate multiple cytokine signals implicated in AD pathogenesis [2]. This chapter offers a comprehensive investigation of the scientific basis, clinical application, safety considerations, and future prospects of JAK inhibitors in the management of atopic dermatitis.

## 2. Overview of atopic dermatitis

### 2.1 Epidemiology and burden of disease

Around 15–20% of children and 2–10% of adults usually suffer from atopic dermatitis worldwide, with increasing prevalence in industrialized nations [3]. Although the disease often starts in early childhood and persists into adulthood, adult-onset AD is also sometimes seen. In terms of the quality of daily life, AD usually causes chronic itchy, visible skin lesions resulting in sleep disturbance, and psychological distress. Also, the disease showed an economic burden directly through increased healthcare costs and indirectly by loss of productivity [3].

### 2.2 Pathogenesis of AD

The pathogenesis of AD includes a multifaceted interaction among epidermal barrier dysfunction, immune dysregulation, and microbial colonization. The process is usually started by genetic mutations, particularly in the filaggrin gene (FLG), affecting the skin barrier integrity resulting in allergen penetration and microbial invasion through skin [4]. As a result, the immune system is activated through type 2 helper T cell (Th2)-mediated responses—leading to the release of pro-inflammatory cytokines including IL-4, IL-13, IL-31, and thymic stromal lymphopoietin (TSLP) [5]. However, the process chronicity is attributed to additional immunological pathways such as Th1, Th17, and Th22 responses. Consequently, the central involvement of cytokine signaling has highlighted the therapeutic potential of targeting intracellular transduction mechanisms, particularly the JAK-STAT pathway in AD [6].

## 3. The JAK-STAT pathway in atopic dermatitis

### 3.1 Structure and function of JAK-STAT Signaling

The JAK-STAT pathway is a primary intracellular signaling mechanism in which a lot of cytokines, growth factors, and hormones employ their effects [7]. The pathway involves four Janus kinase proteins (JAK1, JAK2, JAK3, and TYK2) and seven STAT proteins (STAT1–STAT6). JAKs are usually activated *via* phosphorylation and subsequently recruit and phosphorylate STATs once the ligand binds to surface cytokine receptors. Subsequently, the activated STATs translocate to the nucleus and modulate transcription of immune regulation, inflammation, and cell proliferation genes.

### 3.2 Role in immune dysregulation of AD

In atopic dermatitis, many cytokines can hyperactivate the JAK-STAT resulting in disease pathogenesis. These cytokines include:

DOI: http://dx.doi.org/10.5772/intechopen.1011354

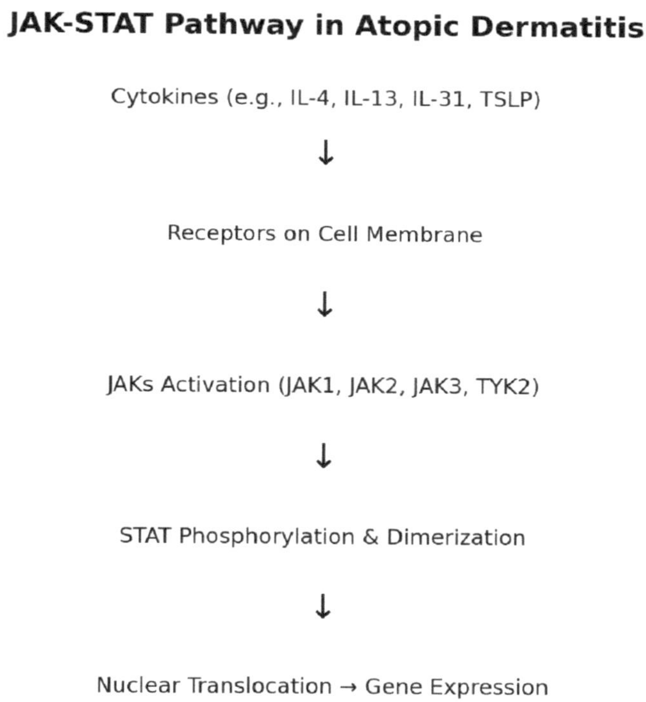


**Figure 1.**
*Schematic representation of the JAK-STAT signaling pathway in atopic dermatitis. This illustration highlights the involvement of cytokines (IL-4, IL-13, IL-31, and TSLP) and their associated JAK kinases, leading to STAT activation and transcription of inflammatory genes (illustrated by the authors).*

- IL-4 and IL-13, the critical mediators of Th2 inflammation, signal *via* JAK1 and JAK3 [8].
- IL-31, responsible for inducing pruritus, signals through JAK1 and JAK2 [8].
- TSLP, which activates dendritic cells and initiates Th2 polarization, also utilizes JAK1 and JAK2 [8].

Given the pathway's central role in amplifying inflammatory signals in AD, JAK inhibitors are considered a strategic therapeutic method to modulate disease activity by disrupting different cytokine cascades simultaneously (**Figure 1**).

## 4. Mechanism of action of JAK inhibitors

### 4.1 Classification: Selective vs. non-selective inhibitors

JAK inhibitors are classified based on their selectivity toward different members of the JAK family:

- Selective JAK1 inhibitors (e.g., upadacitinib, abrocitinib) predominantly block JAK1, which is essential for signaling of pro-inflammatory cytokines such as IL-4, IL-13, and IL-31. These are particularly appropriate in AD due to their central role in Th2-driven inflammation and pruritus [9].

- Pan-JAK inhibitors (e.g., tofacitinib, ruxolitinib) target multiple JAK enzymes simultaneously, resulting in wider immunomodulatory effects but potentially higher risk of complications [10].

- Topical JAK inhibitors, such as ruxolitinib cream, produce localized suppression of the JAK-STAT pathway with minimal systemic absorption, reducing systemic side effects while successfully managing localized lesions [11].

### 4.2 Pharmacokinetics and pharmacodynamics

JAK inhibitors are composed of orally bioavailable small molecules. The onset of action of these agents is usually rapid. These molecules are metabolized primarily by the hepatic pathways, especially cytochrome P450 enzymes. Thus, these drugs should be taken with caution in patients with hepatic impairment or those on interacting drugs. In terms of absorption, topical formulations have negligible systemic absorption. The sublevel plasma concentrations of the drug resulting in minimal systemic effects. JAK inhibitors reduce the transcription of genes associated with inflammation, cytokine release, and pruritus through blocking phosphorylation and activation of STAT proteins. This multitargeted inhibition provides symptom relief among different phases of AD severity [11].

## 5. Clinical evidence and efficacy

### 5.1 Oral JAK inhibitors

Several JAK inhibitors have been assessed in randomized controlled trials (RCTs) for moderate-to-severe atopic dermatitis.

- Upadacitinib, a selective JAK1 inhibitor, showed significant improvement in EASI-75 (Eczema Area and Severity Index—75% improvement) scores as early as week 2, with sustained efficacy through 16 and 52 weeks. In the Measure Up 1 and 2 trials, upadacitinib 30 mg outperformed placebo with a satisfactory pruritus reduction profile [12].

- Abrocitinib, also a selective JAK1 inhibitor, has relieved rapid reduction in itch and skin lesion severity in the JADE trials. JADE MONO-1 and JADE MONO-2 confirmed statistically significant improvement in both EASI and Investigator Global Assessment (IGA) scores within the first month [13].

- Tofacitinib, a pan-JAK inhibitor approved for other autoimmune diseases, has been studied off-label in AD. Although it has approved effectiveness, some concerns regarding its broad immunosuppressive effects and FDA safety warnings have limited its long-term use in dermatology [14].

### 5.2 Topical JAK inhibitors

- Ruxolitinib cream is the first topical JAK inhibitor approved for mild-to-moderate AD. This drug reported significant improvements in both lesion severity and itch relief in comparison with vehicles in the TRuE-AD1 and TRuE-AD2 phase III trials. The favorable safety profile of this drug proved its suitability for long-term intermittent use, especially in sensitive skin areas [15].

### 5.3 Comparative efficacy

JAK inhibitors have a faster onset of action and broader cytokine blockade in comparison with traditional therapies. While biologics like dupilumab target specific cytokines (e.g., IL-4Rα), JAK inhibitors affect multiple signaling pathways [15]. This broad mechanism of action leads to more rapid and complete symptom control. However, this wider immunosuppression may also increase the risk of adverse events, which necessitates individualized treatment decisions by the healthcare providers.

## 6. Safety and tolerability

### 6.1 Adverse events

The most commonly reported adverse events in JAK inhibitor trials include:

- Nasopharyngitis and headache
- Nausea and acne, particularly with oral agents
- Raised creatine phosphokinase (CPK) levels
- Raised liver enzymes
- Herpes zoster reactivation, especially in older adults or those on concomitant immunosuppressive therapy.

Less frequently, venous thromboembolism (VTE) and serious infections have been reported, especially in high-risk populations [16].

These risks are generally dose-dependent and more common with pan-JAK inhibitors or higher doses of selective JAK1 agents.

### 6.2 Monitoring recommendations

To mitigate safety concerns, baseline and periodic monitoring should include:

- Complete blood count (CBC)
- Liver function tests (LFTs)
- Lipid profile
- Tuberculosis screening (prior to initiation)
- Vaccination status (especially varicella-zoster) [17]

While topical ruxolitinib usually does not require close laboratory monitoring due to the limited systemic absorption, a clinical observation remains important.

### 6.3 Risk mitigation strategies

Multiple risk mitigation strategies have been identified for a safer use of these drugs. Careful patient selection and dose adjustments are important strategies. Lower doses may be required for older adults or those with comorbidities. The healthcare providers should use alternative therapies in patients with a history of VTE, malignancy, or serious infections [16].

## 7. Patient selection and clinical use

### 7.1 Indications and criteria for use

Regarding the targeted population, JAK inhibitors are prescribed for patients with moderate-to-severe AD who have not achieved appropriate control with topical therapies or biologics. While oral agents like upadacitinib and abrocitinib are typically used in adolescents and adults, ruxolitinib cream is appropriate for mild-to-moderate disease in patients aged 12 and above [18].

Ideal candidates may include:

- Individuals with the rapid symptom escalation or intense pruritus
- Patients who cannot tolerate injectables (e.g., dupilumab)
- Those with contraindications to biologic therapy
- Patients requiring intermittent oral treatment courses

JAK inhibitors can be used as monotherapy or alongside emollients and topical anti-inflammatories.

### 7.2 Practical prescribing considerations

- Initiation: Evaluate for infection risk, TB exposure, and vaccination history
- Dosing: Start with lowest effective dose, especially in older adults
- Monitoring: Regular laboratory tests (CBC, LFTs, lipids) at baseline and 4–12 week intervals
- Counseling: Discuss risks of immunosuppression, photosensitivity, and shingles

Topical agents may be used for (**Table 1**):

- Facial or intertriginous areas where steroids are prohibited.
- Maintenance therapy in remitting patients.
- Adjunctive treatment during flares.

| Drug | Target JAK(s) | Route | Approval status | Clinical trials | Common AEs |
|---|---|---|---|---|---|
| Upadacitinib | JAK1 | Oral | FDA-approved | Measure Up 1 & 2 | Acne, CPK elevation |
| Abrocitinib | JAK1 | Oral | FDA-approved | JADE MONO 1 & 2 | Nausea, headache |
| Ruxolitinib | JAK1/2 | Topical | FDA-approved | TRuE-AD 1 & 2 | Application site reactions |
| Tofacitinib | JAK1/3 | Oral | Not approved for AD | Early-phase trials | Infection risk |

**Table 1.**
*Summary of JAK inhibitors in atopic dermatitis.*

## 8. Challenges and controversies

### 8.1 Long-term safety concerns

Despite short-term efficacy of JAK inhibitors, some doubts are remaining regarding the long-term use of these drugs. The FDA black box warning (issued in 2021 for tofacitinib and extended to all systemic JAK inhibitors) cites risks for:

- Cardiovascular events
- Malignancy
- Thromboembolism
- Serious infections [19]

Although these concerns originally stem from rheumatoid arthritis studies, caution is needed in dermatology patients, especially those with comorbidities.

### 8.2 Regulatory and access barriers

- Different geographic acceptance and insurance restrictions impact access
- Failure of biologics before JAK inhibitor start are required by some regions.
- Cost and lack of generic formulations also limit wide usage [20].

### 8.3 Real-world use and adherence

Real-world data shows high treatment discontinuation rates, which may be attributed to adverse events or perceived lack of efficacy. The adherence and satisfaction can be improved by better patient education, regular follow-up, and early control of side effects [21].

## 9. Future directions and emerging therapies

### 9.1 Pipeline developments

Ongoing trials are exploring:

- Dual or allosteric JAK inhibitors with greater selectivity

- Topical TYK2 inhibitors, potentially safer for chronic use
- Combination regimens (e.g., JAK inhibitors + biologics) [22]

### 9.2 Biomarker-driven therapy

Biomarkers including serum cytokine profiles and gene expression markers can be included in future personalized treatment plans in order to predict response and decrease side effects [22].

### 9.3 Long-term registries

Currently, large observational studies and registries (e.g., CorEvitas [23], TREAT [24]) are emerging for long-term safety monitoring and effectiveness comparison in different patient populations.

## 10. Conclusion

JAK inhibitors are considered a huge advance in the treatment guidelines of atopic dermatitis [25]. These drugs provide a rapid, targeted, and reversible immunomodulation therapy alternative to the traditional management plans. However, these therapies must be used with caution. Appropriate patient selection, monitoring, and awareness of potential risks are vital for safer drug administration. Currently, JAK inhibitors are becoming a key component in the management of atopic dermatitis as a result of the existing clinical experience advances and long-term evidence. These drugs may be used in conjunction with or even preceding biologics in specific circumstances [26].

## Acknowledgements

The authors acknowledge the use of digital reference management tools for organizing and formatting the references in this chapter. All references were subsequently reviewed and verified manually by the authors.

## Author details

Mohammed Alraddadi[1*], Abdullah Ahmed Alhejaily[1] and Amr Molla[2]

1 Faculty of Medicine, University of Tabuk, Tabuk, Saudi Arabia

2 College Medicine, Taibah University, Madinah, Saudi Arabia

*Address all correspondence to: dr.m.o.alraddadi@gmail.com

## References

[1] Weidinger S, Novak N. Atopic dermatitis. Lancet. 2016;**387**(10023):1109-1122. DOI: 10.1016/S0140-6736(15)00149-X

[2] Tsai HR, Lu JW, Chen LY, et al. Application of Janus kinase inhibitors in atopic dermatitis: An updated systematic review and meta-analysis of clinical trials. Journal of Personalized Medicine. 2021;**11**(4):279. DOI: 10.3390/jpm11040279

[3] Odhiambo JA, Williams HC, Clayton TO, Robertson CF, Asher MI. Global variations in prevalence of eczema symptoms in children from ISAAC phase three. The Journal of Allergy and Clinical Immunology. 2009;**124**(6):1251-1258.e23. DOI: 10.1016/j.jaci.2009.10.009

[4] Palmer CN, Irvine AD, Terron-Kwiatkowski A, et al. Common loss-of-function variants of the epidermal barrier protein filaggrin are a major predisposing factor for atopic dermatitis. Nature Genetics. 2006;**38**(4):441-446. DOI: 10.1038/ng1767

[5] Gittler JK, Shemer A, Suárez-Fariñas M, et al. Progressive activation of TH2/TH22 cytokines and selective epidermal proteins characterizes acute and chronic atopic dermatitis. The Journal of Allergy and Clinical Immunology. 2012;**130**(6):1344-1354. DOI: 10.1016/j.jaci.2012.07.012

[6] Damsky W, King BA. JAK inhibitors in dermatology: The promise of a new drug class. Journal of the American Academy of Dermatology. 2017;**76**(4):736-744. DOI: 10.1016/j.jaad.2016.12.005

[7] Schwartz DM, Bonelli M, Gadina M, O'Shea JJ. JAK inhibition as a therapeutic strategy for immune and inflammatory diseases. Nature Reviews Drug Discovery. 2017;**16**(12):843-862. DOI: 10.1038/nrd.2017.201

[8] Oetjen LK, Mack MR, Feng J, et al. Sensory neurons co-opt classical immune signaling pathways to mediate chronic itch. Cell. 2017;**171**(1):217-228.e13. DOI: 10.1016/j.cell.2017.08.006

[9] Guttman-Yassky E, Teixeira HD, Simpson EL, et al. Once-daily upadacitinib versus placebo in adolescents and adults with moderate-to-severe atopic dermatitis (measure up 1 and measure up 2): Two replicate, double-blind, randomized, placebo-controlled phase 3 trials. Lancet. 2021;**397**(10290):2151-2168. DOI: 10.1016/S0140-6736(21)00588-2

[10] Bissonnette R, Papp KA, Poulin Y, et al. Topical tofacitinib for atopic dermatitis: A phase IIa randomized trial. The British Journal of Dermatology. 2016;**175**(5):902-911. DOI: 10.1111/bjd.14871

[11] Kim BS, Sun K, Papp K, et al. Effects of ruxolitinib cream on pruritus and quality of life in atopic dermatitis: Results from a phase 2, randomized, dose-ranging, vehicle- and active-controlled study. Journal of the American Academy of Dermatology. 2020;**82**(6):1305-1313. DOI: 10.1016/j.jaad.2020.02.009

[12] Simpson EL, Papp KA, Blauvelt A, et al. Efficacy and safety of upadacitinib in patients with moderate to severe atopic dermatitis: Analysis of follow-up data from the measure up 1 and measure up 2 randomized clinical trials. JAMA Dermatology. 2022;**158**(4):404-413. DOI: 10.1001/jamadermatol.2022.0029

[13] Silverberg JI, Simpson EL, Thyssen JP, et al. Efficacy and safety of abrocitinib in patients with moderate-to-severe atopic dermatitis: A randomized clinical trial. JAMA Dermatology. 2020;**156**(8):863-873. DOI: 10.1001/jamadermatol.2020.1406

[14] Winthrop KL. The emerging safety profile of JAK inhibitors in rheumatic disease. Nature Reviews Rheumatology. 2017;**13**(4):234-243. DOI: 10.1038/nrrheum.2017.23

[15] Papp K, Szepietowski JC, Kircik L, et al. Long-term safety and disease control with ruxolitinib cream in atopic dermatitis: Results from two phase 3 studies. Journal of the American Academy of Dermatology. 2023;**88**(5):1008-1016. DOI: 10.1016/j.jaad.2022.09.060

[16] U.S. Food and Drug Administration. Drug Safety Communication: FDA Requires Warnings about Increased Risk of Serious Heart-Related Events, Cancer, Blood Clots, and Death for JAK Inhibitors. 2021. Available from: https://www.fda.gov/drugs/drug-safety-and-availability/fda-requires-warnings-about-increased-risk-serious-heart-related-events-cancer-blood-clots-and-death. [Accessed: August 9, 2025]

[17] Samuel C, Cornman H, Kambala A, Kwatra SG. A review on the safety of using JAK inhibitors in dermatology: Clinical and laboratory monitoring. Dermatologic Therapy. 2023;**13**(5):729-749. DOI: 10.1007/s13555-023-00892-5

[18] Haag C et al. A practical guide to using oral Janus kinase inhibitors for atopic dermatitis from the international eczema council. British Journal of Dermatology. 2025;**92**(1):135-143

[19] Agboola F, Atlas SJ, Brouwer E, Carlson JJ, Hansen RN, Herron-Smith S, et al. JAK inhibitors and monoclonal antibodies for the treatment of atopic dermatitis: Effectiveness and value: A summary from the Institute for Clinical and Economic Review's New England Comparative Effectiveness Public Advisory Council. Journal of Managed Care & Specialty Pharmacy. 2022;**28**(1):108-114. DOI: 10.18553/jmcp.2022.28.1.108

[20] He Q, Xie X, Chen Q, Li W, Song Z, Wang X, et al. Janus kinase inhibitors in atopic dermatitis: An umbrella review of meta-analyses. Frontiers in Immunology. 2024;**15**:1342810

[21] Eichenfield LF, Simpson EL, Papp K, et al. Efficacy, safety, and long-term disease control of ruxolitinib cream among adolescents with atopic dermatitis: Pooled results from two randomized phase 3 studies. American Journal of Clinical Dermatology. 2024;**25**(4):669-683. DOI: 10.1007/s40257-024-00855-2

[22] Tsiogka A, Kyriazopoulou M, Kontochristopoulos G, Nicolaidou E, Stratigos A, Rigopoulos D, et al. The JAK/STAT pathway and its selective inhibition in the treatment of atopic dermatitis: A systematic review. Journal of Clinical Medicine. 2022;**11**(15):4431. DOI: 10.3390/jcm11154431

[23] CorEvitas. CorEvitas Atopic Dermatitis Registry. Available from: https://www.ppd.com/our-solutions/clinical/real-world-data/registries/dermatology/ [Accessed: August 9, 2025]

[24] Bosma AL, Spuls PI, Garcia-Doval I, et al. TREatment of ATopic eczema (TREAT) registry taskforce: Protocol for a European safety study of dupilumab and other systemic therapies in patients with atopic eczema. The British Journal of Dermatology. 2020;**182**(6):1423-1429. DOI: 10.1111/bjd.18452

[25] Ko HC, Woo YR, Ko JY, et al. Consensus-based guidelines for the treatment of atopic dermatitis in Korea (part II): Biologics and JAK inhibitors. Annals of Dermatology. 2025;**37**(4):216-227. DOI: 10.5021/ad.24.154

[26] Monoclonal antibodies and JAK inhibitors in atopic dermatitis – Management guidelines and managed-care considerations. The American Journal of Managed Care. 2024;**30**(12):e439-e448

Chapter 5

# Biologics in the Treatment of Atopic Dermatitis

*Zinah Sharara*

## Abstract

Atopic dermatitis (AD) is a chronic inflammatory skin condition with variable incidence patterns, typically beginning in childhood but following diverse clinical courses. While mild cases respond to topical treatments, such as corticosteroids and calcineurin inhibitors, severe AD traditionally required ultraviolet therapy or conventional immunosuppressants, like ciclosporin and methotrexate. Recent therapeutic advances have introduced targeted biologics and Janus kinase inhibitors, marking significant progress in AD management.

**Keywords:** atopic dermatitis (AD), eczema, biologic therapies, monoclonal antibodies, targeted therapy, dupilumab

## 1. Introduction

Atopic dermatitis (AD) is considered a prevalent chronic inflammatory skin disease that imposes a significant strain on patients' quality of life and healthcare systems. It encompasses a complex pathogenesis involving microbial imbalance, compromised skin barrier integrity, and immune system changes, which manifest in a variety of clinical presentations [1]. The therapeutic strategy for AD has been reformed by acknowledging the crucial role of type 2 inflammatory pathways, opening the doors for targeted immunological treatments.

The treatment options for patients with moderate-to-severe AD have improved significantly in recent years. Several targeted therapies are now approved by the European Medicines Agency (EMA), including four biologic agents: dupilumab (IL4Rα antagonist approved in 2017), tralokinumab (IL13 antagonist, approved in 2021), lebrikizumab (IL13 antagonist, approved in 2023), and, most recently, nemolizumab (IL31Rα antagonist, approved in 2024) [2]. Moreover, three oral Janus kinase (JAK) inhibitors are introduced, which have a role in the regulation of intracellular signaling cascades. These innovative therapeutic modalities represent a significant addition to the treatment armamentarium, contributing to improved disease management and patients' quality of life.

## 2. Approved biologics

### 2.1 Dupilumab

#### *2.1.1 Mechanism of action and regulatory approval*

Dupilumab (Dupixent®) is the first biologic therapy approved for treating atopic dermatitis (AD) in adults. The Food and Drug Administration (FDA) granted approval for dupilumab on March 28, 2017. In the UK, it was authorized on 1st of August 2018 for adult patients with moderate and severe AD who have not shown a response at best to one other systemic treatment such as methotrexate, azathioprine, ciclosporin, or mycophenolate mofetil, or when none of the immunosuppressants are tolerated [3, 4]. It was also approved in 2020 for patients aged ≥6 years with moderate-to-severe AD. Additionally, in 2020, dupilumab received approval for use in patients aged 6 years and older with moderate-to-severe AD [5].

Dupilumab is an IgG monoclonal antibody with high affinity binding to interleukin-4 alpha subunit receptor (IL-4), thereby blocking the pathways of IL-4 and IL-13, important type 2 inflammatory signaling cytokines [6].

#### *2.1.2 Clinical use and administration*

Dupilumab is used in Europe for several conditions, namely: moderate-to-severe AD, moderate-to-severe prurigo nodularis, asthma (adjuvant maintenance treatment), nasal polyps (as adjuvant), chronic rhinosinusitis, and eosinophilic esophagitis [7].

Adults typically begin Dupilumab with 600 mg, injected subcutaneously as two injections of 300 mg, then to maintain treatment as 300 mg every 2 weeks. Body weight is taken into consideration when treating children and adolescents, and the dose can vary. Patients who have both asthma and eczema may receive different dosing regimens tailored to their conditions [8].

#### *2.1.3 Clinical trials outcome*

The efficacy of dupilumab in patients with moderate-to-severe atopic dermatitis was assessed *via* two Phase 3 monotherapy trials, placebo-controlled, SOLO1, and SOLO2. These trials enrolled a total of 671 patients who received subcutaneous injection of 300 mg dupilumab given weekly or every other week for a total of 16 weeks [9]. Results demonstrated that complete or almost complete clearance of symptoms was achieved in 36% of dupilumab-treated patients, a stark contrast to only 9% of those receiving placebo. The primary outcome was reached in the SOLO1 trial by 38% in patients on dupilumab every other week and 37% in the dupilumab weekly dosing group, compared to a 10% response in the placebo. SOLO2 showed similar efficacy with 36% of dupilumab-treated group hitting the primary endpoint against 8% in the placebo. These outcomes assert dupilumab's significant symptom improvement in patients with moderate-to-severe atopic dermatitis [10].

#### *2.1.4 Drug retention analysis: Dupilumab vs. standard systemic treatments in atopic dermatitis*

The extracted data from the registry of BioDay involving 402 dupilumab-treated patients were compared to cohorts on cyclosporine (356 patients) or methotrexate

(89 patients). Dupilumab had significantly higher drug survival rates at the first and second years (91 and 88%, respectively), far surpassing cyclosporine (37 and 20%), and methotrexate (41 and 33%). These differences were statistically significant, indicating dupilumab's superior persistence and patient retention relative to conventional systemic agents [11].

The LIBERTY AD CHRONOS study has investigated dupilumab combined with standard topical steroid or topical calcineurin inhibitors for 52 weeks. Moderate and severe eczema patients have been treated with dupilumab 300 mg injection weekly or every 2 weeks versus placebo alongside topical therapies [12].

At the 16-week mark, 39% of dupilumab recipients achieved (IGA 0/1) clear or nearly clear skin, as compared to 12% of the placebo group. Additionally, 64% (weekly) and 69% (bi-weekly) of adults reached at least 75% improvement in the EASI-75 index, as compared to 23% improvement in the placebo group. The improvement was continuous until the 52 weeks [12].

Long-term data of more than 5 years extracted from the LIBERTY AD extension trial showed a persistent effect with a total of 2677 treated adults who showed improvement in EASI of at least 75% at 88.9% [13].

### *2.1.5 Laboratory and clinical safety profile*

Laboratory data analyses from the SOLO1, SOLO2, and CHRONOS trials demonstrated no significant changes in the laboratory basic markers among the dupilumab and placebo groups. Importantly, dupilumab treatment was not associated with clinically meaningful lab abnormalities, suggesting that routine laboratory monitoring is unnecessary in typical clinical use [14]. Both conjunctivitis and reactions at the injection site were frequently reported with dupilumab, showing a durable efficacy and acceptable safety profile when used with topical treatments [12].

### *2.1.6 Real-world efficacy*

An explorative real-world study reported substantial improvements in disease severity over time. The mean EASI scores dropped significantly in week 16. Moreover, after 2 years of permanent treatment, EASI scores further reached 1.73, demonstrating sustained clinical benefits [15].

A total of 3303 patients have received subcutaneous weekly 300 mg doses of dupilumab for 16 weeks. All data were included in A meta-analysis that analyzed a total of 22 controlled randomized trials, which revealed a mean EASI score reduction of 69.6%. These findings reinforce that dupilumab is a tolerable and highly efficient option for moderate and severe atopic eczema [16].

Another meta-analysis of 17 studies up to April 2024 further confirmed that dupilumab improves eczema symptoms and highly enhances Dermatology Life Quality Index (DLQI) [17].

Dupilumab has shown significant improvement in chronic hand eczema across various subtypes, with good safety, significant effectiveness, and tolerability [18].

### *2.1.7 Safety and effectiveness of dupilumab in children*

Dupilumab has also been studied in children between 6 months up to the age of 6 years old. In a phase 2 trial, pediatric patients received a single dose of 3 mg per Kg, which achieved EASI reductions of 44.6%, and another dose tested, 6 mg per kg of body weight; the Drop in EASI was 49.7% after 3 weeks. Older children showed slightly better responses. By the fourth week, responses diminished mostly in the lower dose group [19]. The real-life data from 80 children aged 6–11 years with moderate-to-severe atopic dermatitis treated with dupilumab for 3 months showed a significant decrease in disease severity scores including SCORAD and IGA (0/1). This supports dupilumab's effectiveness and safety in this pediatric population [20].

## 2.2 Tralokinumab

### *2.2.1 Overview and mechanism of action*

Tralokinumab (Adtralza®) is a monoclonal IgG4 antibody that selectively neutralizes IL-13, a key cytokine linked to the aetiopathogenesis of moderate-to-severe atopic dermatitis (AD) [21]. Tralokinumab works by binding to IL-13, preventing its interaction with the IL-13 receptors on cutaneous cells. This interruption blocks downstream signaling pathways that trigger inflammation and skin barrier dysfunction. By this mechanism, tralokinumab mitigates the inflammatory symptoms of AD and restores the barrier function.

IL-13 levels correlate closely with disease severity [21–23]. It drives inflammation, negatively impacts skin-barrier function, resulting in filaggrin and loricrin down-regulation, and increases type II inflammation by raising levels of eosinophils and activating T cells [9]. Additionally, IL-13 compromises the cutaneous defense through lowering the production of keratinocyte antimicrobial peptide, hence increasing risks of *Staphylococcus aureus* colonization and infections [24, 25].

### *2.2.2 Regulatory approval and clinical use*

Tralokinumab has been authorized by major regulatory organizations. The European Commission, the UK's Medicines and Healthcare products Regulatory Agency, and the US Food and Drug Administration approved the medication for the treatment of patients with moderate-to-severe eczema who fail to respond to topical treatment and qualify for systemic modalities. This approval was based on findings from phase 3 clinical studies (ECZTRA 1, 2, and 3), which demonstrated notable skin clearance, symptom reduction, pruritis alleviation, and overall improvement in quality of life. Generally, safety levels comparable to a placebo [26].

The standard dosing regimen is subcutaneous injections, starting with a 600 mg subcutaneous loading dose, then treatment is maintained with 300 mg every 2 weeks [26].

### *2.2.3 Safety and real-world effectiveness*

Tralokinumab has shown strong real-world effectiveness and a satisfactory safety profile in managing moderate and severe atopic dermatitis, especially among patients without prior systemic treatments. Over a 24-week period, it significantly improved clinical indices such as the EASI and pruritus scores, while reducing key inflammatory biomarkers [27].

Common reported side effects of tralokinumab were upper respiratory tract infections and conjunctivitis; however, tralokinumab was considered with an appropriate safety profile, in a mirroring pattern to placebo in both studies.

A recent multicenter, prospective trial was performed involving adult atopic dermatitis (AD) patients who were 18 years old and older, and who were managed with tralokinumab from July 2021 to August 2023. Reported adverse events (AEs) were mild (58.1%). The most common AEs were eye disorders (28.6%), general disorders, such as malaise (9.5%), nervous system disorders, such as headache (9.5%), and skin/subcutaneous disorders, such as hair loss (9.5%). Although eye disorders were the most frequent, 66.7% of these cases were mild and rarely caused treatment discontinuation [28].

#### *2.2.4 Clinical trial outcomes*

A phase III trial compared the response between patients receiving tralokinumab injections of 300 mg each two times a week and a placebo, where patients also used topical corticosteroids for 16 weeks, at least 56.0% of the treatment group achieved EASI (EASI-75) versus 35.7% of the placebo. Moreover, the IGA (0/1) score showed a significant improvement in the treatment group versus the placebo. Both parameters have been maintained well until week 32 [29].

ECZTRA 1 and ECZTRA 2 are phase III trials assessing adults suffering from moderate-to-severe AD who were randomized into group 1, who received tralokinumab injections of 300 mg every 2 weeks versus placebo for a total of 52 weeks. Tralokinumab-treated patients significantly responded at week 16, as both scores (EASI-75 and IGA 0/1) have improved for both ECZTRA 1 and ECZTRA 2. Most responders have maintained improvements to week 52 with continued treatment without additional therapies [30].

A phase IIb study combining tralokinumab with topical glucocorticoids showed significant improvements after 12 weeks in EASI, Scoring Atopic Dermatitis (SCORAD), Dermatology Life Quality Index (DLQI), and pruritus compared to placebo. Among adverse events that were reported, upper respiratory tract infections were the most common emergent [31].

Another phase II, a 30-week trial in which tralokinumab was administered over 16 weeks, the dose was 300 mg every 2 weeks, demonstrated that the medication did not impair immune responses to either meningococcal or tetanus/diphtheria/pertussis (TDP) vaccines, confirming a favorable safety profile consistent with phase 3 studies [32].

Tralokinumab has proven effective in real-world settings, and 65.5% of responders achieved a 50% improvement in EASI (EASI-50) and experienced enhanced quality of life without serious adverse events reported [33].

### **2.3 Lebrikizumab**

#### *2.3.1 Overview and mechanism of action*

Lebrikizumab is a humanized antibody with anti-IL-13 effect. Preventing the activation of IL-4Rα and IL-13Rα1, a crucial part in signal transduction in inflammation, thus decreases symptoms of atopic dermatitis (AD) [34, 35].

#### *2.3.2 Regulatory approval and clinical use*

Lebrikizumab (Ebglyss®) was recommended by NICE for patients aged 12 and over, who are not improving or cannot tolerate systemic immunosuppressants. The medication has gained approval in 2023 from the European Commission and the UK MHRA [36, 37].

### *2.3.3 Dose and administration*

Lebrikizumab is administered *via* the subcutaneous route, an initial dose of 500 mg, then maintained with 250 mg every 2 weeks for 16 weeks. Good responders can then receive 250 mg every 4 weeks, while a partial responder can have 250 mg/per 2 weeks with possible extension until the 24th week, then switching to every 4 weeks [38].

### *2.3.4 Clinical trials and effectiveness*

In the phase III trials, which assessed lebrikizumab as a monotherapy and when combined with topical steroid therapies, in the treatment of eczema, lebrikizumab-treated group demonstrated a significant improvement compared to placebo [39].

In the Advocate 1 and 2 studies, which evaluated the effect of lebrikizumab in patients with moderate-to-severe dermatitis, the main goal was specified as having symptom-free or almost symptom-free skin after week 16. Secondary objectives were a substantial reduction in eczema severity and improvements in pruritus and sleep quality. About one-third of patients receiving lebrikizumab reached the primary goal, compared to roughly 10–13% in the placebo group. Major improvement in eczema severity was achieved in 50% in lebrikizumab-treated group, while this was seen in around 16–18% of placebo patients. The need for additional rescue treatment was similar in both studies, affecting around 14–16% of patients [40].

Lebrikizumab-treated patients improved significantly in a dose-dependent pattern by week 16, with the highest dose showing the greatest reduction in the severity. This improvement was also accompanied by a rapid response of pruritis [41, 42].

Mild-to-moderate adverse effects were reported in treatment subjects and had not caused treatment to stop. Generally, the medication was tolerable and a low proportion of conjunctivitis and reactions at the site of injection were noticed [41, 43].

## **2.4 Nemolizumab**

Nemolizumab suppresses signal transduction between IL-31 and the α-subunit of the IL-31 receptor, which eventually improves pruritis and regulates barrier function [42], as well as prevent the fibrosis in prurigo nodularis [44].

### *2.4.1 Regulatory approval and clinical use*

Nemolizumab (Nemluvio)® was approved BY EMA in February 2025 for the management of moderate-to-severe AD in patients older than 12-year-old [45] provided as a 30 mg monthly injection.

### *2.4.2 Clinical trials and effectiveness*

ARCADIA 1 and ARCADIA 2 are phase III, placebo-controlled trials that evaluated Nemolizumab in patients aged 12 years with moderate-to-severe eczema. These studies involved treating 1142 patients with nemolizumab who were advised to maintain topical steroid application and 586 patients with a placebo combined with topical steroid therapy. The primary endpoints were set as improvement of IGA 0/1 with a $\geq$ 2-point improvement from baseline and EASI75 improvement at week 16 [46]. Both primary endpoints were achieved at the end of 16 weeks of treatment. The nemolizumab-treated group attained 36 and 38% improvement in IGA 0/1 versus the quarter of the placebo group. EASI 75 also notably improved in nemolizumab-treated group by 44 and 42% which is more significant than the placebo group, for which EASI 75 was reached by 29 and 30%.

Another phase III, a randomized and placebo-controlled study; 60 mg nemolizumab monthly subcutaneous injections administered subcutaneously up to 16 weeks; during which topical steroid treatment was allowed. Both the mean decrement in EASI and the mean pruritis score improved in the nemolizumab treatment group. EASI showed a significant reduction at week 16 for nemolizumab group (42.8%) as compared to the placebo group (21.4%) [47].

In regard to adverse effects in the clinical trials of nemolizumab in AD and prurigo nodularis, the following were reported often: injection site reaction, nasopharyngitis, upper respiratory tract infections, and type 1 hypersensitivity reactions, including mild urticaria and angioedema [45, 47, 48]. Notably, none has caused treatment discontinuation.

## 3. Therapies undergoing research in AD

### 3.1 Etokimab (ANB020)

Etokimab is a humanized monoclonal antibody that antagonizes IL-33, a significant cytokine in type 2 inflammation and highly expressed in the skin of atopic patients with active disease. It acts by provoking IL-4, IL-5, and IL-13. It also promotes mast cell degranulation in the process of triggering Th2 and ILC2 [49].

Etokimab was evaluated in a phase II, a proof-of-concept trial, showing significant improvements in Dermatology Life Quality Index (DLQI), itch scores (SCORAD), Investigator Global Assessment (IGA) 0/1, and EASI equated to placebo. However, in the ATLAS (phase IIb trial), 300 patients with moderate to severe atopic eczema were evaluated for 16 weeks; none of the etokimab-treated group with different regimens met the primary endpoint (ClinicalTrials.gov Identifier: NCT03533751) [50].

In another recent (Phase II) trial, 302 adults with moderate-to-severe AD were evaluated, and etokimab was reported ineffective in meeting the end point, in which (ClinicalTrials.gov Identifier NCT 03533751) [51].

### 3.2 Fezakinumab

Fezakinumab is a monoclonal antibody with an anti-IL-22 effect. It was reported to be effective in the phase IIa trial as compared to placebo, especially in patients with severe dermatitis with high IL-22 levels [52].

### 3.3 Tezepelumab

Tezepelumab is a monoclonal antibody that binds to an inflammatory cytokine called thymic stromal lymphopoietin linked to the pathophysiology of atopic dermatitis. Tezepelumab was evaluated in a phase IIa clinical trial (ClinicalTrials.gov Identifier NCT02525094). Numerical improvements were reported beyond placebo scores, and primary endpoints scores were met at week 12, which further improved in week 16; however, changes were not statistically significant over the placebo group [53].

## 4. OX40 and OX40L axis blockers

OX40 and its ligand, OX40L, act as secondary costimulatory molecules, increasing T cell responses. The nuclear factor κB1 and phosphoinositide 3-kinase/protein kinase B pathways are activated by this interaction, thus promoting proliferation, survival, and differentiation of effector T cells. These signaling cascades trigger the production and reactivation of long-term immune responses *via* activation of memory T cells.

1. *Telazorlimab* (ISB 830/GBR 830) is a humanized monoclonal antibody antagonize OX40 receptor. Telazorlimab was evaluated in a two-part trial (ClinicalTrials.gov Identifier NCT03568162) and reported substantial and progressive score improvement in patients with moderate and severe dermatitis [54].

2. *Rocatinlimab* (KHK4083) is a fully humanized monoclonal antibody that antagonizes OX40 receptors. A phase II trial resulted in an improvement of EASI, which was maintained statistically significant from the baseline up to 16 weeks [55]. At present, Rocatinlimab is under further phase III trials [51].

3. *Amlitelimab* is IgG4 monoclonal antibody antagonize OX40L. The effectiveness has been evaluated in two phase II trials (ClinicalTrials.gov identifier NCT05131477) [56]. It was administered at various doses, significantly reduced eczema severity (EASI scores) in comparison with placebo in adults with severe atopic dermatitis over 24 weeks. Clinical improvements were maintained up to 52 weeks, even for many patients who stopped treatment, with sustained biomarker reductions and were well tolerated

## 5. Conclusion

The three approved biologics for the management of atopic dermatitis are dupilumab, tralokinumab, and nemolizumab. Several biologics are undergoing phase II and phase III trials targeting the cytokines involved in type 2 inflammation. Given the unmet demands from the patient's perspective, using these drugs has the potential to influence the atopic march as well as other comorbidities. Although biologics are very well tolerated, their benefit-to-risk ratio is a crucial challenge for pharmacovigilance. More studies are therefore needed to evaluate their safety and effectiveness.

## Conflict of interest

The authors declare no conflict of interest.

*DOI: http://dx.doi.org/10.5772/intechopen.1013012*

## Author details

Zinah Sharara
National Health Service (NHS), Community Dermatology Clinics
(Health Harmonie), UK

*Address all correspondence to: zinah.sharara@healthharmonie.co.uk

## References

[1] Yew YW, Thyssen JP, Silverberg JI. A systematic review and meta-analysis of the regional and age-related differences in atopic dermatitis clinical characteristics. Journal of the American Academy of Dermatology. 2019;**80**:390-401

[2] Royeck S. Biologics in the treatment of atopic dermatitis: Approved active substances and monoclonal antibodies in advanced clinical trials. Allergo Journal International. 5 Aug 2025:1-8

[3] Selondonccg.nhs.uk. Atopic Dermatitis – Dupilumab Pathway. London, UK: South East London Clinical Commissioning Group; 2022. Available from: https://selondonccg.nhs.uk/wp-content/uploads/dlm_uploads/2021/09/Atopic-dermatitis-%E2%80%93-dupilumab-pathway-FINAL-June-2021.pdf [Accessed: July 20, 2025]

[4] Nice.org.uk. Dupilumab for Treating Moderate to Severe Atopic Dermatitis. Technology Appraisal Guidance (TA534). London, UK: National Institute for Health and Care Excellence; 2018. Available from: https://www.nice.org.uk/guidance/ta534/resources/dupilumab-for-treating-moderate-to-severe-atopic-dermatitis-pdf-82606900940485 [Accessed: July 10, 2025]

[5] Müller S, Maintz L, Bieber T. Treatment of atopic dermatitis: Recently approved drugs and advanced clinical development programs. Allergy. 2024;**79**(6):1501-1515

[6] Guttman-Yassky E, Bissonnette R, Ungar B, Suárez-Fariñas M, Ardeleanu M, Esaki H, et al. Dupilumab progressively improves systemic and cutaneous abnormalities in patients with atopic dermatitis. Journal of Allergy and Clinical Immunology. 2019;**143**(1):155-172

[7] European Medicines Agency. Dupixent: EPAR - European Public Assessment Report [Internet]. Amsterdam, The Netherlands: European Medicines Agency; 2025. Available from: https://www.ema.europa.eu/en/medicines/human/EPAR/dupixent [Accessed: August 25, 2025]

[8] European Medicines Agency. EMA-Approval Dupixent. Available from: https://www.ema.europa.eu/en/medicines/human/EPAR/dupixent [Accessed: August 27, 2025]

[9] Thaçi D, Simpson EL, Beck LA, Bieber T, Blauvelt A, Papp KA, et al. Efficacy and safety of dupilumab monotherapy in adults with moderate-to-severe atopic dermatitis: A pooled analysis of two phase 3 randomized trials (SOLO 1 and SOLO 2). Journal of the American Academy of Dermatology. 2019;**80**(2):359-370.e9. DOI: 10.1016/j.jaad.2018.10.043

[10] Simpson EL, Bieber T, Guttman-Yassky E, Beck LA, Blauvelt A, Cork MJ, et al. Two phase 3 trials of dupilumab versus placebo in atopic dermatitis. New England Journal of Medicine. 2016;**375**(24):2335-2348

[11] Spekhorst LS, Ariëns LF, van Der Schaft J, Bakker DS, Kamsteeg M, Oosting AJ, et al. Two-year drug survival of dupilumab in a large cohort of difficult-to-treat adult atopic dermatitis patients compared to cyclosporine a and methotrexate: Results from the BioDay registry. Allergy. 2020;**75**(9):2376

[12] Blauvelt A, de Bruin-Weller M, Gooderham M, Cather JC, Weisman J,

Pariser D, et al. Long-term management of moderate-to-severe atopic dermatitis with dupilumab and concomitant topical corticosteroids (LIBERTY AD CHRONOS): A 1-year, randomised, double-blinded, placebo-controlled, phase 3 trial. The Lancet. 2017;**389**(10086):2287-2303

[13] Beck LA, Bissonnette R, Deleuran M, Nakahara T, Galus R, Coleman A, et al. Dupilumab in adults with moderate to severe atopic dermatitis: A 5-year open-label extension study. JAMA Dermatology. 2024;**160**:805-812

[14] Wollenberg A, Beck LA, Blauvelt A, Simpson EL, Chen Z, Chen Q, et al. Laboratory safety of dupilumab in moderate-to-severe atopic dermatitis: Results from three phase III trials (LIBERTY AD SOLO 1, LIBERTY AD SOLO 2, LIBERTY AD CHRONOS). The British Journal of Dermatology. 2020;**182**(5):1120-1135. DOI: 10.1111/bjd.18434

[15] Song D, Gong WP, Xiao GL. Comparative analysis of the efficacy of abrocitinib and dupilumab in the treatment of atopic dermatitis. Clinical, Cosmetic and Investigational Dermatology. 31 Dec 2025:817-825

[16] Halling AS, Loft N, Silverberg JI, Guttman-Yassky E, Thyssen JP. Real-world evidence of dupilumab efficacy and risk of adverse events: A systematic review and meta-analysis. Journal of the American Academy of Dermatology. 2021;**84**(1):139-147

[17] Sun Y, Liu H, Gao Y, Sang H, Kong Q. Effects of dupilumab on quality of life in patients with atopic dermatitis: A systematic review and meta-analysis of randomized controlled trials. Frontiers in Pharmacology. 2025;**16**:1587977

[18] Lee A. Beyond the itch: Emerging therapies for chronic hand eczema. Journal of Dermatology for Physician Assistants. 1 Jul 2025;**19**(3):36

[19] Paller AS, Siegfried EC, Simpson EL, Cork MJ, Lockshin B, Kosloski MP, et al. A phase 2, open-label study of single-dose dupilumab in children aged 6 months to <6 years with severe uncontrolled atopic dermatitis: Pharmacokinetics, safety and efficacy. Journal of the European Academy of Dermatology and Venereology : JEADV. 2021;**35**(2):464-475. DOI: 10.1111/jdv.16928

[20] Lasek A, Bellon N, Mallet S, Puzenat E, Bursztejn AC, Abasq C, et al. Effectiveness and safety of dupilumab in the treatment of atopic dermatitis in children (6-11 years): Data from a French multicentre retrospective cohort in daily practice. Journal of the European Academy of Dermatology and Venereology. 2022;**36**(12):2423-2429

[21] Newsom M, Bashyam AM, Balogh EA, Feldman SR, Strowd LC. New and emerging systemic treatments for atopic dermatitis. Drugs. 2020;**80**(11):1041-1052. DOI: 10.1007/s40265-020-01335-7

[22] Wollenberg A, Blauvelt A, Guttman-Yassky E, Worm M, Lynde C, Lacour JP, et al. Tralokinumab for moderate-to-severe atopic dermatitis: Results from two 52-week, randomized, double-blind, multicentre, placebo-controlled phase III trials (ECZTRA 1 and ECZTRA 2). British Journal of Dermatology. 2021;**184**(3):437-449

[23] European Medicines Agency. CHMP/559383/2017. Imraldi: EPAR - European Public Assessment Report [Internet]. Amsterdam, The Netherlands: European Medicines Agency; 2017. Available from: https://www.ema.europa.eu/en/documents/assessment-report/imraldi-epar-public-assessment-report_en.pdf [Accessed: April 25, 2025]

[24] Bieber T. Interleukin-13: Targeting an underestimated cytokine in atopic dermatitis. Allergy. 2020;**75**(1):54-62

[25] Tsoi LC, Rodriguez E, Degenhardt F, Baurecht H, Wehkamp U, Volks N, et al. Atopic dermatitis is an IL-13–dominant disease with greater molecular heterogeneity compared to psoriasis. Journal of Investigative Dermatology. 2019;**139**(7):1480-1489

[26] Popovic B, Breed J, Rees DG, Gardener MJ, Vinall LM, Kemp B, et al. Structural characterisation reveals mechanism of IL-13-neutralising monoclonal antibody tralokinumab as inhibition of binding to IL-13Rα1 and IL-13Rα2. Journal of Molecular Biology. 20 Jan 2017;**429**(2):208-219

[27] Hagino T, Onda M, Saeki H, Fujimoto E, Kanda N. Effects of tralokinumab on clinical and laboratory indexes in atopic dermatitis: A 24-week real-world study. Dermatitis. 2025;**36**(3):235-243

[28] Hagino T, Uchiyama A, Kosaka K, Araki T, Saeki H, Fujimoto E, et al. Transition of blood biomarkers during 24-week treatment with lebrikizumab or tralokinumab in atopic dermatitis: A real-world analysis stratified by prior systemic therapy. Dermatitis. Jul 2025;**27**(4):e10-e97

[29] Silverberg JI, Toth D, Bieber T, Alexis AF, Elewski BE, Pink AE, et al. Tralokinumab plus topical corticosteroids for the treatment of moderate-to-severe atopic dermatitis: Results from the double-blind, randomized, multicentre, placebo-controlled phase III ECZTRA 3 trial. British Journal of Dermatology. 2021;**184**(3):450-463

[30] Wollenberg A, Blauvelt A, Guttman-Yassky E, Worm M, Lynde C, Lacour JP, et al. Tralokinumab for moderate-to-severe atopic dermatitis: Results from two 52-week, randomized, double-blind, multicentre, placebo-controlled phase III trials (ECZTRA 1 and ECZTRA 2). The British Journal of Dermatology. 2021;**184**(3):437-449. DOI: 10.1111/bjd.19574

[31] Wollenberg A, Howell MD, Guttman-Yassky E, Silverberg JI, Kell C, Ranade K, et al. Treatment of atopic dermatitis with tralokinumab, an anti-IL-13 mAb. The Journal of Allergy and Clinical Immunology. 2019;**143**(1):135-141

[32] Merola JF, Bagel J, Almgren P, Røpke MA, Lophaven KW, Vest NS, et al. Tralokinumab does not impact vaccine-induced immune responses: Results from a 30-week, randomized, placebo-controlled trial in adults with moderate-to-severe atopic dermatitis. Journal of the American Academy of Dermatology. 2021;**85**(1):71-78

[33] Sebastian N, Chircop O, Clayton TH, Kreeshan FC, Hunter HJ, Warren RB. Real-World clinical experience of tralokinumab in a tertiary centre: An alternative for patients with conjunctivitis on dupilumab? Dermatology and Therapy. 29 May 2025:1-5

[34] May RD, Fung M. Strategies targeting the IL-4/IL-13 axes in disease. Cytokine. 2015;**75**(1):89-116

[35] Ultsch M, Bevers J, Nakamura G, Vandlen R, Kelley RF, Wu LC, et al. Structural basis of signaling blockade by anti-IL-13 antibody lebrikizumab. Journal of Molecular Biology. 2013;**425**(8):1330-1339

[36] Keam SJ. Lebrikizumab: first approval. Drugs. 2024;**84**(3):347-353

[37] Almirall SA. NICE Recommends Ebglyss (Lebrikizumab) for Use in

Moderate to Severe Atopic Dermatitis in the NHS England in Eligible Adolescents and Adults. Barcelona, Spain: Almirall SA; 2024. Available from: https://www.almirall.com/newsroom/news/nice-recommends-ebglyss-lebrikizumab-for-use-in-moderate-to-severe-atopic-dermatitis-in-the-nhs-england-in-eligible-adolescents-and-adults-1 [Accessed: August 27, 2025]

[38] European Medicines Agency. EMA Approval of Ebglyss [Internet]. Amsterdam, The Netherlands: European Medicines Agency. Available from: http://www.ema.europa.eu/en/medicines/human/EPAR/ebglyss [Accessed: August 27, 2025]

[39] Thaci E. Efficacy and safety of Lebrikizumab is maintained up to three years in patients with moderate-to-severe atopic dermatitis: ADvocate 1, ADvocate 2, and ADjoin long term extension trial. In: 2024 European Academy of Dermatology and Venereology Congress. 25 Sep 2024

[40] Silverberg JI, Guttman-Yassky E, Thaçi D, Irvine AD, Gold SL, Blauvelt A, et al. Two phase 3 trials of Lebrikizumab for moderate-to-severe atopic dermatitis. The New England Journal of Medicine. 2023;**388**:1080-1091

[41] Simpson EL, Gooderham M, Wollenberg A, Weidinger S, Armstrong A, Soung J, et al. Efficacy and safety of lebrikizumab in combination with topical corticosteroids in adolescents and adults with moderate-to-severe atopic dermatitis: A randomized clinical trial (ADhere). JAMA Dermatology. 2023;**159**(2):182-191

[42] Nakashima C, Otsuka A, Kabashima K. Interleukin-31 and interleukin-31 receptor: New therapeutic targets for atopic dermatitis. Experimental Dermatology. 2018;**27**(4):327-331

[43] Guttman-Yassky E, Blauvelt A, Eichenfield LF, Paller AS, Armstrong AW, Drew J, et al. Efficacy and safety of lebrikizumab, a high-affinity interleukin 13 inhibitor, in adults with moderate to severe atopic dermatitis: A phase 2b randomized clinical trial. JAMA Dermatology. 2020;**156**(4):411-420

[44] European Commission. Information for Healthcare Professionals. Nemluvio [Internet]. Brussels, Belgium: European Commission; 2025. Available from: https://ec.europa.eu/health/documents/communityregister/2025/20250212165149/anx_165149_de.pdf

[45] Nemolizumab for treating moderate to severe atopic dermatitis in people 12 years and over. In: NICE Guidance [Internet]. London: National Institute for Health and Care Excellence; 2025. Available from: https://www.nice.org.uk/guidance/ta1077 [Accessed: August 22, 2025]

[46] Silverberg JI, Wollenberg A, Reich A, Thaçi D, Legat FJ, Papp KA, et al. Nemolizumab with concomitant topical therapy in adolescents and adults with moderate-to-severe atopic dermatitis (ARCADIA 1 and ARCADIA 2): Results from two replicate, double-blind, randomised controlled phase 3 trials. The Lancet. 2024;**404**(10451):445-460

[47] Kabashima K, Matsumura T, Komazaki H, Kawashima M. Trial of nemolizumab and topical agents for atopic dermatitis with pruritus. New England Journal of Medicine. 2020;**383**(2):141-150

[48] Ständer S, Yosipovitch G, Legat FJ, Reich A, Paul C, Simon D, et al. Efficacy and safety of nemolizumab in patients

with moderate to severe prurigo nodularis: The OLYMPIA 1 randomized clinical phase 3 trial. JAMA Dermatology. 2025;**161**(2):147-156

[49] Chen YL, Gutowska-Owsiak D, Hardman CS, Westmoreland M, MacKenzie T, Cifuentes L, et al. Proof-of-concept clinical trial of etokimab shows a key role for IL-33 in atopic dermatitis pathogenesis. Science Translational Medicine. 2019;**11**(515):eaax2945

[50] AnaptysBio. AnaptysBio Reports Etokimab ATLAS Phase 2b Clinical Trial Results [Internet]. San Diego, CA, USA: AnaptysBio, Inc.; 2023. Available from: https://ir.anaptysbio.com/news-releases/news-release-details/anaptysbio-reports-etokimab-atlas-phase-2b-clinical-trial [Accessed: September 10, 2024]

[51] Lo Y, Cheng TT, Huang CJ, Cheng YC, Chyuan IT. Advancing therapeutic strategies in atopic dermatitis: Emerging targets and personalized approaches. Biomolecules. 2025;**15**(6):838

[52] Guttman-Yassky E, Brunner PM, Neumann AU, Khattri S, Pavel AB, Malik K, et al. Efficacy and safety of fezakinumab (an IL-22 monoclonal antibody) in adults with moderate-to-severe atopic dermatitis inadequately controlled by conventional treatments: A randomized, double-blind, phase 2a trial. Journal of the American Academy of Dermatology. 2018;**78**(5):872-881

[53] Simpson EL, Parnes JR, She D, Crouch S, Rees W, Mo M, et al. Tezepelumab, an anti–thymic stromal lymphopoietin monoclonal antibody, in the treatment of moderate to severe atopic dermatitis: A randomized phase 2a clinical trial. Journal of the American Academy of Dermatology. 2019;**80**(4):1013-1021

[54] Rewerska B, Sher LD, Alpizar S, Pauser S, Pulka G, Mozaffarian N, et al. Phase 2b randomized trial of OX40 inhibitor telazorlimab for moderate-to-severe atopic dermatitis. Journal of Allergy and Clinical Immunology: Global. 2024;**3**(1):100195

[55] Guttman-Yassky E, Simpson EL, Reich K, Kabashima K, Igawa K, Suzuki T, et al. An anti-OX40 antibody to treat moderate-to-severe atopic dermatitis: A multicentre, double-blind, placebo-controlled phase 2b study. The Lancet. 2023;**401**(10372):204-214

[56] Weidinger S, Blauvelt A, Papp KA, Reich A, Lee CH, Worm M, et al. Phase 2b randomized clinical trial of amlitelimab, an anti-OX40 ligand antibody, in patients with moderate-to-severe atopic dermatitis. Journal of Allergy and Clinical Immunology. 2025;**155**(4):1264-1275